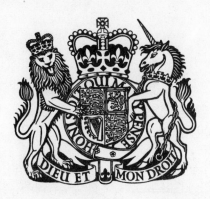

Report of the Committee of Enquiry into Mental Handicap Nursing and Care

Chairman: PEGGY JAY

Volume I

*Presented to Parliament by the Secretary of State
for Social Services, the Secretary of State for Scotland
and the Secretary of State for Wales
by Command of Her Majesty*
March *1979*

LONDON
HER MAJESTY'S STATIONERY OFFICE
£3.00

Cmnd. 7468-I

D1425349

ISBN 0 10 174680 6

ii

MEMBERS OF THE COMMITTEE

Mrs Peggy Jay — (Chairman)

Mr N Bosanquet — Lecturer in Economics, The City University

Mr J B Cottrell — Divisional Nursing Officer, Stoke Park Group of Hospitals, Bristol. (Formerly Divisional Nursing Officer, Hensol Hospital, Glamorgan)

Miss M Faulds — Senior Lecturer (Social Work), Paisley College of Technology. (Formerly Director of Social Work, Inverness County)

Mr T A Foster — Director of Social Services, Metropolitan Borough of Tameside

Mr A Hunt — Director of Social Services, Hampshire

Miss M Ingham* — Head of Ida Darwin Hospital School

Dr G Kerr — Consultant Psychiatrist and Medical Administrator, Dovenby Hall Hospital, Cumbria

Mr N Lees — Area Nursing Officer, Derbyshire Area Health Authority

Mr H McCree — District Nursing Officer, Winchester and Central Hampshire Health District

Councillor W Merritt — Formerly Chairman, Social Services Committee, Association of Metropolitan Authorities

Mrs B Nicolas — Education Officer, General Nursing Council for England and Wales

Professor M R Olsen — Professor of Social Work, Birmingham University, (Formerly Senior Lecturer, University College of North Wales)

Dr D Ricks — Consultant-in-Charge Children's Department, Harperbury Hospital. Hon. Consultant in Mental Handicap, Departments of Paediatrics and Child Psychiatry, University College Hospital

Mr D Thomas — Principal Clinical Psychologist, Northgate Hospital, Northumberland Area Health Authority

Mr D O Williams — Chairman, Staff Side, General Whitley Council for the Health Services

Mrs J M Williams — Deputy Director and Senior Lecturer in Social Studies, Department of Extra Mural Studies, University of Birmingham

Mr D Williamson — Senior Tutor, Lennox Castle Hospital, Glasgow

Miss P H F Young — Director, Central Council For Education and Training in Social Work

SECRETARY

Mr D Dufton — Department of Health and Social Security

*Retired from Committee October 1977

CHAIRMAN'S PREFACE

TO:
The Rt Hon David Ennals, MP
Secretary of State for Social Services

The Rt Hon Bruce Millan, MP
Secretary of State for Scotland

The Rt Hon John Morris, QC, MP
Secretary of State For Wales

Dear Secretaries of State

On behalf of the Committee of Enquiry into Mental Handicap Nursing and Care I have the honour of submitting our report to you.

We have seen our appointment and the ensuing 3 years' work as a logical and inevitable reflection of mounting public concern about the quality of life being experienced by mentally handicapped adults and children in residential care. A major aspect of this concern has been the conditions in which some mental handicap nursing staff are working.

Our Committee was established following the recommendations in the report of the Briggs Committee on Nursing in which the whole question was raised of the logic of having two separate forms of staff training and recruitment to meet the needs of mentally handicapped people in hospital or local authority care. Our terms of reference did not allow us to consider the structure of residential services, or to make recommendations about who should provide them, but we did interpret our remit as covering consideration of the conditions in which our newly trained staff would work. We have built up our recommendations on the actual needs of mentally handicapped people and the staff who care for them. These we have reached through our questionnaire to all staff organisations; through a survey conducted by the OPCS for our Committee; through oral evidence and finally through the visits and work experience of our widely based membership.

We are convinced that change is not only necessary but inevitable; in addition to the Briggs proposals there is the 1971 White Paper which set the trend for development of locally based services for mentally handicapped people. We recognise that a doubling of the workforce will cost money. The acute need for additional finance will not be in the NHS sector but rather for local authorities where the setting up of a specific fund to launch the new training scheme will be crucial.

We were given a challenging task which was enormously eased by the quality of the members of the Committee all of whom have served in their personal capacity and not as representatives of organisations. I express my gratitude to them. Despite heavy professional commitments of their own they have given generously of their time in attendance and travelling. The wide base of the Committee membership has enabled us to draw on current work experience at many levels of the health and local authority services. It is noteworthy that with their widely disparate backgrounds members have found themselves in broad agreement not only on the need for change but on the direction of change.

It will be observed that the two notes of personal reservation at the end of our report refer to methods by which these changes should be achieved, and not to the changes themselves. In the case, however, of the minority report by David Williams the Committee find themselves in profound disagreement not only with the methods but also with the objectives of change advocated which, it should be said, are contradictory to the terms of the White Paper. Nevertheless these contributions will add to the relevance and quality of the debate which will inevitably follow the publication of this paper. Debate there must be, but we hope that it will be brought to a speedy conclusion.

Finally our warmest thanks are due to our Secretary Denis Dufton whose hard work, sense of humour, experience and diplomatic skills have been of the greatest value in our discussions. Our thanks are also due to Ursula Brennan and Joan McCoy who have assisted Mr Dufton and the Committee in innumerable ways. Our gratitude must also be recorded to Elisabeth Woods, Assistant Secretary, DHSS, Norman Hill and Stella Earl, DHSS Nursing Officers, Christiana Horrocks and Ruth Sanders, Social Work Services Officers of the Department, Paul Wilson of OPCS and to our nurse observers from Scotland, Wales and Northern Ireland.

It has been said that nothing will be the same again for mentally handicapped people or the staff who work with them after the publication of our report. We commend our work to you in the belief that nothing should be the same. Change there must be. We hope it will be on the lines of our recommendations.

Yours sincerely,

PEGGY JAY

CONTENTS

VOLUME 1

CHAPTER 4: MANPOWER

CHAPTER 5: STAFF TRAINING

CHAPTER 6: ORGANISATION AND MANAGEMENT

CHAPTER 7: FINANCE AND PRIORITIES

LIST OF FIGURES

PEN PICTURES OF MENTALLY HANDICAPPED PEOPLE

Who are the mentally handicapped people in need of care? We have tried to keep before us at all times an image of the very disparate group of people who are classed together as "the mentally handicapped." All our deliberations have had as their starting point the individuals who are the clients for residential services. We prepared the five pen pictures which follow as fictitious examples to illustrate some of the wide range of problems which are coped with every day by mentally handicapped people and those who care for them.

1. JILL BROWN

Jill, her mother's third child, was delivered by forceps after a prolonged labour. At birth she was limp and pale, did not cry and needed resuscitating in a special unit so her mother did not see her immediately. When she left hospital she was fretful and difficult to feed, moving very little and hardly responding to her mother's voice or face. Her worried mother was told that her brain had been damaged which made her apprehensive when she picked Jill up or handled her, although she was an experienced mother. As she grew older she became more stiff and was unable to sit or reach out and was extremely difficult to feed. However, she was quite a friendly responsive child, although her mother had to take care not to startle her because she would so readily cry and go into spasm. She was unable to help her mother dress her, once her legs and arms became stiff. She was unable to sit on her own and had to be helped into standing and she could not move around on her own with support as normal toddlers would begin to do. Her physical handicap became more and more evident although she was a little girl who gave great pleasure because she smiled readily, had a lively expression, and although not speaking made noises to show she was pleased or excited. Now, aged 8, she is sitting with a better posture in her own wheelchair and able to make some attempt at feeding herself though her aim of the spoon is poor and she cannot load it; she helps dress herself, putting one arm into a sleeve, but needs to be helped with washing and feeding, and is incontinent. She attends a special school which she greatly enjoys and is clearly popular with the staff; she tries hard with matching tasks and constructive toys and enjoys music, particularly in the company of other children. Although they find the school staff very reassuring, her parents worry about her slow progress and as she gets bigger and heavier they become increasingly anxious about their own capacity to cope with her in the future.

2. JACK GREEN

Jack was his mother's first child; she was unwell during her pregnancy but carried on working full-time, eventually needing to be admitted to hospital for a rest until Jack was born. From the start he was a fretful baby with an unpredictable sleeping pattern so that his parents found him very wearying. They both noticed that he paid little attention to them although he could obviously hear because he would startle and cry lustily at an unusual or loud noise and would look around him though his gaze was fleeting and rarely fixed on his mother's face. At a few months old they were alarmed because he occasionally jerked his arms, stiffened and looked blank. He was seen in the

xiii

local hospital children's department where various tests were carried out; he was then started on medicine and within a few weeks the attacks stopped. For several months afterwards he seemed lethargic and uninterested but gradually became more active and alert though with the same undiscriminating interest in the world around him. He was sitting up on his 1st birthday though it took two more years before he could walk. Throughout this time he followed an aimless repetitive play with any object to hand and seemed resistant to efforts made by his parents to teach him to wash or dress or feed. He was obviously capable of these actions but seemed unaware of the purpose of any self-help, resented attempts made to direct his activity and lapsed readily into his simple play. Although quite vocal he did not babble nor use any words but gradually learned what was expected of him by becoming accustomed to a routine. His parents discovered that he could be shown how to do things by putting his hands or arms through the actions rather than by telling him and that he fairly quickly learned what to expect: he would, for instance, fetch his coat before going out, or get up to the table when his meal was prepared. As he became more mobile his management became increasingly difficult. He was nimble and very active, climbing on furniture; he could use his hands very efficiently but tended to use this skill in unfastening or dismantling things so that the household furniture and fittings had to be adapted to withstand his exploratory play. The main worries were his high level of activity, his apparently unintentional destructive ability, and his complete unawareness of danger; he would run into the road or climb on top of a shed with a speed and imperviousness to reprimand which made watching him closely a constant worry. Understandably his parents became very concerned to find a playgroup but he was beyond the scope of several which they tried. They found themselves resorting to special activities to calm him down or keep him occupied such as riding in the car or playing on the swings in the local park. They were greatly relieved when he was admitted to the nearby special school where the staff seemed much more accepting of his behaviour. With their help he gradually learned to feed more efficiently and, on a good day, would dress himself. He began imitating some simple words though he did not use them appropriately and remained wilful and impetuous. He is now an affectionate responsive boy though his parents find his care exhausting.

3. JOHN SMITH

No-one realised that John was handicapped until he went to a secondary school. Until then he had been a quiet boy and although he did not do well at lessons his parents were not worried by this. They had both left school early and did not place great importance on learning. When he changed schools at 11 he soon became very upset and frightened and would not go to school. His mother asked for help and John was found to have an intelligence quotient of 70. His parents readily agreed that he should go to a special school in the same town because it had a good reputation for helping children and was housed in an attractive old mansion.

John flourished there and was regarded as one of the cleverer boys. His mother became an active member of the parents' group at the school. He left at 16 and began work immediately as a labourer in a local concern. He is 34 and still works in the same job which pays well. He lives with his parents who are now retired. His life has changed very little in the past 18 years. He works regularly, is a keen and successful fisherman and his mother not only looks after his creature comforts but has always been the family scribe and negotiator. Neither John nor his father have ever had to deal with the family affairs or public officials. She does it all.

John has recently started going to a local disco and his parents are worried because he is no longer saving money and has had two accidents in his car. They wonder where this new behaviour is going to lead and are trying to understand that perhaps he has grown up a little later than his contemporaries. His father and mother are now nearing 70 and their health is poor. John will find life complicated and more difficult when he no longer has their protection.

4. JEAN FORBES

Jean Forbes was born in 1944 and was admitted to hospital in that year. Her family history has not been documented. Today Jean appears totally incapable of being communicated with. She evinces no interest in her environment, has no curiosity, and is unaware of care staff unless they approach her too closely.

Although she is able and encouraged to walk Jean spends most of her time sitting in a chair, rocking back and forth, plucking the skin of her face or sucking and biting her hands. At frequent intervals she engages in lengthy bouts of high pitched screaming and, at these times, she will bite, scratch or kick those who approach to pacify her. Occasionally she will rise from her chair and smash a window on impulse, to her own injury.

All efforts to modify her behaviour have ended in failure and Jean remains resistant to being fed. If, on the other hand, food is placed before her she will gulp it down so quickly that regurgitation inevitably follows. At other times she will chew her clothing or soft toys, gnaw the side of her chair and, since she is doubly incontinent, if the opportunity arises she will daub herself with faeces.

Jean appears to have some appreciation of music. For example, if dance music is being played she will stop rocking momentarily and move her head from side to side rhythmically, but although the other residents will dance and sing she does not join or mimic them.

Over the years considerable effort has been directed towards stimulating Jean, both physically and mentally. It would appear that she has an innate fear of physical contact and simple activities such as changing her clothing, bathing, brushing her hair, or attending to minor injuries sustained in her outbursts, meet with noisy and violent resistance.

Dedicated care staff have sought to establish a one-to-one relationship with Jean, using every means and technique at their disposal—music, mobiles, pets, toys and, most of all, affection—all to little avail.

5. JOSEPH EVANS

Joseph Evans was born in 1933 of normal parents. His father was a Joiner and his mother a Post-Mistress. He has two elder brothers and a younger sister, all professional people.

Joseph enjoyed good health and was a happy, active child until he contracted measles at the age of 2 years. Complications followed which left Joseph blind, deaf, mute and paralysed. His parents were unable to cope with the problems of caring adequately for the child and he was admitted to hospital in 1936. He has been confined to bed since his original illness. Nevertheless, he is well-nourished, his skin is intact and he is the recipient of care and concern from all members of the caring team.

Although he receives physiotherapy regularly, Joseph has developed contractures of his lower limbs, no doubt caused by his many years of inactivity. Because of his posture, feeding poses difficulties and care staff have proved themselves ingenious in developing techniques of feeding which allow him to enjoy a varied and adequate diet.

The extent of his disabilities has necessarily limited any communicative ability which Joseph may have. After a meal he makes gentle gurgling noises; other than that he is totally lacking in any response. Care staff take great pride in their day-to-day work with Joseph, chatting to him as they change his bed and attend to his basic needs. His general health is relatively good and with such care there is every probability that Joseph will attain a normal life span.

CHAPTER 1 – INTRODUCTION

APPOINTMENT AND METHOD OF WORK

Appointment

1. On 26 February 1975 the Secretary of State for Social Services, the Rt Hon Mrs Barbara Castle, MP announced the establishment of an enquiry into mental handicap nursing and care under the chairmanship of Mrs Peggy Jay. Our Committee was set up to consider an important recommendation of the Briggs Committee that "a new caring profession for the mentally handicapped should emerge gradually".[1] This recommendation caused lively interest and some controversy among workers in the field of mental handicap, particularly mental handicap nurses. During the conferences and seminars which ensued it became apparent that not only were there divergent views about the needs of mentally handicapped people but also about what was meant by "a new caring profession". Continuing public and political concern together with professional controversy led to the establishment of : (1) the National Development Group, (2) the Development Team and (3) this Committee. Our terms of reference were:

> "To consider recommendation 74 of the Report of the Committee on Nursing (Briggs Committee), in particular to enquire into the nursing and care of the mentally handicapped in the light of developing policies, to examine the roles and aims of nurses and residential care staff required by the health and personal social services for the care of mentally handicapped adults and children; the inter-relationship between them and other health and personal social services staff; how existing staff can best fulfil these roles and aims; in the interest of making the best use of available skills and experience, the possibilities of the career movement of staff from one sector or category to another; the implications for recruitment and training; and to make recommendations."

Terms of Reference

2. It is important to state at the outset that our terms of reference caused us considerable difficulty; our problems were reflected in the widely differing interpretations of our remit which we found on our visits and in the written and oral evidence which we received. Our terms of reference included the very broad injunction "to enquire into the nursing and care of the mentally handicapped" but went on to focus more narrowly on the "roles, aims and skills" of the professional staff required to provide residential services for mentally handicapped people. We debated whether a remit to conduct our enquiry "in the light of developing policies" meant that we must completely avoid an examination of, and recommendations on, "policy", or whether we were simply being asked to show a sensitivity towards national strategies and organisational structures, without necessarily accepting the conceptual and empirical assumptions behind those policies. Many members argued that it would be impossible to examine care and the training and deployment of staff without looking at complementary issues of setting, organisation and resources.

---

1. Numbers in the text refer to the list of references on page 182.

3.   To resolve our difficulties we formulated a number of ground rules. We agreed that the "developing policies" referred to were those outlined in the White Paper "Better Services for the Mentally Handicapped"[2]. We accepted that for the foreseeable future the majority of residential services for mentally handicapped people would continue to develop bilaterally under the management of health and social services authorities. We considered that it was not within our remit to examine whether either health authorities or social services authorities should assume responsibility for all mental handicap residential services, or whether a separate new agency should be established. We did, however, feel strongly that it was a central part of our remit to look at the essential nature of the task of caring for mentally handicapped people, without being constrained by how that task is currently allocated between particular professions or agencies. We also accepted that this "model building" approach might well challenge basic assumptions in or behind current policy and might, if accepted, require subsequent revision of these policies. We also considered that whilst our main focus would be residential care this could not be understood, particularly in relation to children, except in relationship to care within the family. Finally, we think it will be clear from our report that we were convinced that organisational and manpower issues had to be tackled alongside training if our recommendations were to have any validity, credibility and, ultimately significant impact on the quality of care of mentally handicapped people.

Meetings

4.   We met in full session on 31 occasions, including 3 weekend residential meetings, but excluding a number of days devoted to oral evidence. Much of our detailed work was undertaken in Sub Committees, twelve of which were appointed during the life of our Committee.

Visits

5.   We felt that we could not carry out our work effectively in isolation, without seeing for ourselves some of the situations in which care is given. Representative groups of members therefore made numerous visits to hospitals, homes and day centres throughout England, Scotland and Wales. Although our membership contained a fair range of expertise in most of the areas of interest to us these visits provided an opportunity for members to take a closer look at both new and familiar situations. But most important of all they gave staff the opportunity of talking to us and putting to us their ideas for the future organisation and training of their professions. They took full advantage of this opportunity and we are grateful for the trouble and time they took to present their views. A list of the places we visited is at Appendix C.

Evidence

6.   A vital part of any Committee's information-gathering process is the taking of evidence, both written and oral. Towards the end of 1975 we announced that we were ready to receive written evidence, and several thousand copies of a questionnaire were distributed. A copy of this questionnaire is at Appendix A. The questionnaire sought views on the tasks and roles of nurses and local authority residential care staff, and on manpower development. We were particularly anxious that every member of staff concerned with the care of mentally handicapped people should be aware of our existence and purpose

and should know that they could submit evidence, either individually or collectively. In the event a total of 613 separate pieces of evidence were received, ranging from single page letters to long, closely argued papers. A list of written evidence received is at Appendix B. Many of the submissions presented by organisations have been published.

7.   In addition we spent a great deal of time listening to oral evidence. The individuals and organisations presenting oral evidence are also shown in Appendix B. We are grateful to all those who gave evidence, both oral and written, for the contribution which they made to our thinking about mental handicap care.

Research

8.   To supplement the information which we obtained by calling for written evidence, taking evidence orally, and visiting a sample of hospitals and homes we commissioned a study by the Office of Population Censuses and Surveys. This survey covered both factual information and attitudes of staff in mental handicap residential establishments and provided a more up-to-date and wider profile than was currently available of both the staff and the people they were looking after. The survey was conducted on a sample basis and the results were used to provide national indicators. The survey is published as Volume II of this report. We would have liked to commission other research as we felt that we could, as a Committee, have identified a small number of very specific short life projects which would have provided us with useful information. This was not possible as no allocation of funds for this purpose had been made to the Committee. Consequently we had to make do with existing research, which, for the most part, provided a very limited empirical base for deliberations of the kind we had been asked to undertake.

BACKGROUND TO OUR ENQUIRY

The Scope of the Problem

9.   Before we could decide how many and what type of residential care staff* were required we needed to know the prevalence of mental handicap. We needed information on mental handicap, analysed by such factors as age, sex, type and degree of mental handicap, any additional handicaps, place of residence etc. We also needed to know the recent trends in these figures and what factors may influence them, now and in the future, so as to affect short and long term plans. There are however numerous difficulties both in obtaining and in interpreting these figures. In the first place prevalence rates are usually calculated on the basis of use of services. This is not a satisfactory method of calculation for various reasons, for example: existing services may not meet all the demand; an individual may not contact the health, education or social services authority if a particular service is known to be either not available or over subscribed locally; there may be a small number of individuals who do not know of the services available and who are themselves unknown to the

---

*Throughout our Report we have (unless otherwise stated) use the term "residential care staff" to signify all those who are employed in the residential care of mentally handicapped people, whether in the NHS or the local authority social services, including existing mental handicap nurses and existing local authority mental handicap residential care staff. Similarly the term "residential care" is intended to include care in a mental handicap hospital as well as care in a local authority home.

authorities; some mildly mentally handicapped people may be using general social services and may not be identified as mentally handicapped. It is not enough to know how many people are mentally handicapped, we also needed to know something about the degree of handicap. Here we come up against the problem of definition. Mild mental handicap covers a wide range of people from the borderline with severe handicap to the borderline with those whose intelligence is below normal but for whom this does not present a problem. For practical purposes an Intelligence Quotient of 50 is commonly taken as the broad dividing line between mild and severe mental handicap and the IQ range 50–70 is usually used to classify people with mild mental handicap. But such divisions take no account of emotional development, social competence, and environmental and educational influences which affect the functioning of any individual.

10.   Even when the figures have been collected the problem of interpretation remains. It is not possible to say that a certain type of handicap always requires a certain type of service, so that planning and forecasting must be matters of judgement. Ideas about the care needs of mentally handicapped people are constantly changing – in recent years particularly, as residential care staff have begun to discover the hidden potential of their clients – but today's buildings, reflecting yesterday's theories, will limit and define the scope of tomorrow's services. It is therefore particularly important to be flexible and open-minded about ways in which care can be provided and about the extent of the need for different types of care. At present it is generally agreed that some severely handicapped people will require lifelong residential care but there are differences of view across the spectrum of mental handicap in relation to the variety of residential, day and domiciliary services which could or should be provided. In these circumstances it is difficult to estimate the demand for these services and therefore also the staffing required to run them. In the absence of any other figures we have had to use the planning figures set out in the 1971 White Paper which gave projections of numbers of adults and children requiring various types of residential care, hospital treatment, education and day services over the next 15–20 years. But even these figures were tentative and will need to be adjusted in the light of experience. All these constraints mean that the statistics quoted in the following paragraphs have to be interpreted with caution. Futhermore it is likely that preventive measures will reduce the number of children born with mental handicap in future years. The lack of firm figures is not however as damaging to planning as it may appear. In Chapter 4 we explain that a large increase in staffing is necessary and authorities can therefore continue to plan to increase both services and staffing in the foreseeable future without any fear of over provision.

11.   The White Paper, published in 1971, estimated that there may be about 120,000 severely mentally handicapped people in England and Wales, of whom about 50,000 are children. Case register studies over the past 15 years have suggested prevalence rates for severe mental handicap among children varying between 2.95 and 5.81 per thousand population; Figure 1 gives details from some of the major studies.

Figure 1 – PREVALENCE OF SEVERE MENTAL HANDICAP

CASE REGISTER	AGE GROUP	PREVALENCE/1000 POPULATION	
Wessex, 1964	15–19	3.54	– urban
	15–19	3.84	– rural
Camberwell, 1972	5–9	4.39	} urban
	10–14	4.17	
Salford, 1973	5–9	5.73	} urban
	10–14	5.81	
Sheffield, 1975	5–9	2.95	} urban/rural
	10–14	4.65	

References 3–5.

The 10–14 and 15–19 age groups are regarded as the most reliable for measuring the extent of severe mental handicap since most individuals will have been identified by these ages. A large proportion of mentally handicapped people in hospital also have physical handicaps and/or behaviour difficulties which may cause them to function at a lower level than their apparent degree of intellectual handicap would warrant.

12.   Information about the prevalance of the additional incapacities associated with mental handicap can be obtained from a variety of censuses and surveys. The Department of Health and Social Security carried out a "Census of Mentally Handicapped Patients in Hospital in England and Wales at the end of 1970".[6] This produced detailed results on the sex and age; degree of mental handicap; legal status; time spent in hospital; level of intelligence; education, training and employment; visiting; and associated incapacities of the residents. The census showed that a high proportion of the hospital residents had additional incapacities, but that the prevalence of most (though not all) such incapacities reduced with the increasing age of the residents. As might be expected the prevalence of each incapacity was considerably greater among the severely handicapped residents than among the mildly mentally handicapped residents. The prevalence of the various incapacities is shown in Figure 2. A similar census was carried out on mentally handicapped people in local authority and voluntary residential accommodation, in 1970.[7] This provided information on levels of dependency as determined by the residents' self care capacities. As expected, in the majority of local authority homes there were few residents who were appreciably or heavily dependent. The most heavily dependent of local authority residents were in the children's homes rather than the adults' homes. (The disabilities found in these two surveys would not necessarily be permanent.) Our own OPCS survey also provided information about the dependency of hospital and home residents. This information is shown in Figure 3.

13.   The results of the two censuses show that the community services are not yet providing for the significant number of people who would be able to transfer from hospital to the community if places were available, as distinct from people who need an alternative to the family home. The results also suggest that younger less handicapped people are more "acceptable" for residential care in the community than are older, more severely handicapped people. The high proportion of people in community residential care who are of low dependency – and should in theory be able to live in unstaffed accommodation – is probably a reflection of the policies of previous years when large numbers of mentally handicapped people were brought up in institutions regardless of their abilities.

5

FIGURE 2 – INCAPACITIES OF HOSPITAL RESIDENTS, 1970 CENSUS

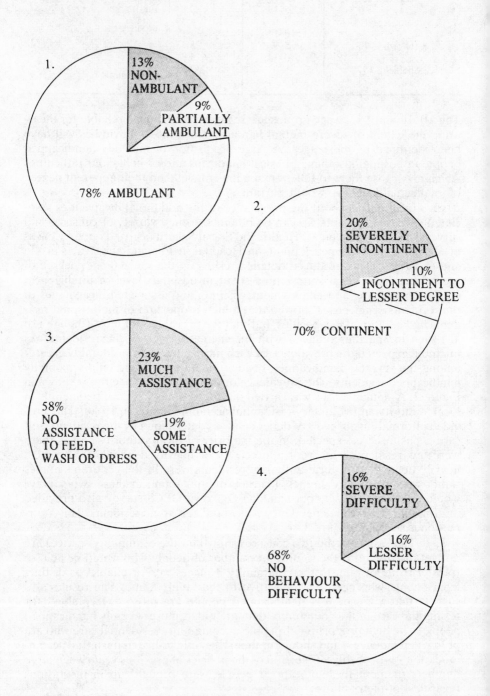

FIGURE 2 – INCAPACITIES OF HOSPITAL RESIDENTS, 1970 CENSUS
(continued)

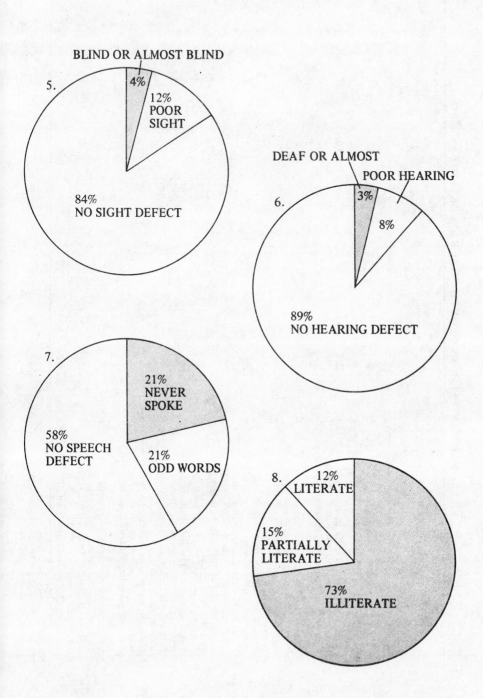

FIGURE 3 – THE EXTENT OF SPECIFIED PHYSICAL ILLNESSES AND HANDICAPS

Proportion of the patients and residents who:	All wards*	All homes†	Adult homes high ability	Adult wards high ability	Adult wards average ability	Adult wards low ability	Adult wards non-ambulant with very low ability	Children's homes	Children's wards
	%	%	%	%	%	%	%	%	%
were blind (or partially sighted)	5	2	2	2	4	7	14	4	11
were deaf (and could not use a hearing aid)	4	2	2	4	4	5	4	3	5
suffered from cerebral palsy (spasticity) ..	14	5	4	4	7	16	67	10	28
suffered from cerebral palsy and were bedridden or had difficulty walking up stairs	12	2	1	3	5	12	67	4	25
suffered from a heart condition	5	3	2	5	5	6	5	4	4
suffered from a heart condition and were bedridden or had difficulty walking upstairs	2	1	1	2	2	2	4	0	2
suffered from asthma, bronchitis or any other respiratory illness	6	7	5	4	6	5	8	17	10
suffered from asthma, bronchitis or any other respiratory illness and were bedridden or had difficulty in walking upstairs	2	1	1	1	2	2	5	1	6
suffered from arthritis	2	1	2	2	2	2	3	0	0
suffered from arthritis and were bedridden or had difficulty walking upstairs	1	1	1	1	1	1	2	0	0
suffered from epilepsy (including controlled epileptics) ..	29	13	12	18	27	36	52	18	44
had at least one epileptic fit in the previous year	19	8	7	10	17	24	33	12	33
had at least one epileptic fit in the previous month	11	5	4	7	9	14	20	8	18
needed a special diet for health reasons ..	8	3	3	7	6	6	17	4	9
were confined indoors on the previous weekday because of a physical illness ..	2	1	1	1	2	2	5	1	3
Base for percentages:									
Total number of patients (reweighted) ..	8,441	1,760	1,416	2,983	2,699	1,347	742	325	673

*Excluding acute sickness wards.
†Excluding homes with 3 or more residents who were not mentally handicapped.
Source: OPCS Survey Table 28.

8

14.   From the foregoing it can fairly be said that mental handicap can be assessed only in terms of a combination of: (a) degree of specific ability and handicap, (b) social competence, (c) level of intelligence and (d) living environment. It is however important to remember that mentally handicapped people do not form a homogeneous group.

Present Provision for Mental Handicap

15.   Figures 4 and 5 below illustrate some of the recent trends in the health and social services. The figures show the developing shift from health service to local authority provision and the reduction in residential places for children. The increase in the allocation of short stay beds is an acknowledgement of the changing rôle expected of hospitals and the number of beds allocated for shortstay use is likely to continue increasing. The totals in Figure 4 do not include the associated day care, training and out patient facilities which mental handicap hospitals provide, or the specialist services for additional handicaps. Figure 5 shows that the independence and variety of living situations offered by unstaffed homes is slowly being recognised. The provision of occupation and training places shows substantial improvement, with current efforts concentrating on special units for the more severely handicapped. Other services in the community – such as sheltered workshops and day care for the under 5s – though not provided primarily for mentally handicapped people also make a contribution to services in this field.

FIGURE 4 – NHS PROVISION (ENGLAND, SCOTLAND AND WALES)

	1970	1974	1975	1976
NHS Residents – adults and children	65,326	60,154	59,119	58,516
NHS Residents – children under 15	7,384	5,666	5,295	4,879
Provision of short-stay beds*	–	701	–	1,080

*England and Wales only. Short-stay residents also included under NHS Residents.
Sources: "In-Patient Statistics from the Mental Health Enquiry for England" (DHSS).
"DHSS: Facilities of Mental Handicap Hospitals and Units – National and Regional Summaries for England".
"Health and Personal Social Services Statistics for Wales" (Welsh Office).
"Scottish Health Statistics" (SHHD).

FIGURE 5 – LOCAL AUTHORITY AND VOLUNTARY PROVISION (ENGLAND AND WALES)

	1970	1977
Places in LA homes—adults and children	5,221	10,158
Places in LA homes—children under 16	1,407	1,721†
Places in LA unstaffed homes	85‡	653
Places in Adult Training Centres	26,649	40,369
Adult Training Centres—places in special care units	§	1,672
Places in voluntary and private homes	1,814*	3,404

§Not available.
*England only.
†Some places were "lost" in the transfer of a number of children's homes to education authorities following the 1970 Education (Handicapped) Children Act.
‡Figure from "The Census of Residential Accommodation: 1970" DHSS.
Sources: "Mental Health Statistics" (DHSS).
"Personal Social Services: Local Authority Statistics" (DHSS and Welsh Office).

16. Figure 5 shows that voluntary and private homes, including communities with facilities for occupation and training, provide a significant proportion of places for mentally handicapped people. In addition, other mentally handicapped adults are living in lodgings and adults and children are living in other kinds of local authority, private or voluntary residential accommodation not specifically designated for mentally handicapped people: for example children may be living with foster parents, or in community homes. The major areas of provision identified here are not intended to delineate the total range of services being used by mentally handicapped people; individuals may be catered for by any of the agencies or organisations providing services for the general public.

The Family

17. Any review of present provision must take into account the important fact that the great majority of mentally handicapped people live at home with their families. (The White Paper of 1971 estimated that 80 per cent of severely handicapped children and 40 per cent of severely handicapped adults, together with most mildly handicapped people lived at home. The present position may, however, be different.) In considering the scope of the problem of providing services account must be taken of the immeasurable support and experience, as well as physical care and control, given within the family to mentally handicapped members living at home. The vulnerability of the family to the problems of mental handicap is not necessarily related to the degree of handicap or the level of dependency of the individual. It is within the family that the overriding need for helping the mentally handicapped person to live as normal a life as possible starts and it continues throughout the different phases of the individual's life. The contribution of families is not fully recognised by those who plan and provide residential care. This has led us to set down (in Chapter 3) the guiding principles of care which should apply wherever mentally handicapped people have resort to services outside their own families.

The Historical Perspective

18. Having considered our client group and the services currently available to that group, we thought it important to look briefly at how the present pattern of service provision came about. In the ensuing paragraphs we provide our outline of the ideas and events which have shaped public and professional attitudes to mental handicap.

The National Health Service – 1948

19. When the National Health Service came into being in 1948 the existing institutions and prevailing public attitudes were the product of the policies and prejudices of the previous 200 years. Over this period of time policies on mental handicap were subject to regular and radical alteration, reflecting the ideas, motives and ideologies of the time; prejudice on the other hand remained constant. The facilities provided were thus often the result of historical accident rather than the product of a rational assessment of the needs of the community. In 1948 mentally handicapped adults were, for the most part, housed in the special public asylums provided by mental deficiency authorities under the 1886 Idiots Act, or in Public Assistance (formerly Poor Law) institutions; in Scotland they were housed in institutions operated by local

authorities under the Local Authority (Scotland) Act 1929. Mentally handicapped children might be similarly placed or, where there was a lesser degree of handicap, might attend special schools or classes provided by local education authorities. Community care, under supervision, was regarded as an appropriate alternative to institutional care, but was not much used by local authorities. The Board of Control, successor to the Lunacy Commissioners, still existed although central control of mental deficiency institutions in England was vested in the Ministry of Health. A survey in 1949 showed that the 53 mental deficiency colonies or state hospitals in operation were staffed by nurses who held the certificate of the Royal Medico-Psychological Association, nurses on the Register of the General Nursing Council, and untrained nursing assistants. A few psychiatric social workers and untrained social workers were operating a form of after-care for discharged patients and for mentally handicapped people in the community, but this activity was confined to areas where the local authority was enthusiastic. Generally in 1948 the experts believed that people suffering from mental handicap deserved more than a life of confinement, regimentation and idleness and that education and training were necessary (even if some were pessimistic about the likelihood of much improvement in the patient's condition). But this attitude had not always prevailed and professional attitudes had been through many sometimes conflicting phases before arriving at this consensus.

Changing Attitudes

20. One of the earliest known references to mental handicap is a 14th century statute which distinguishes "born fools" (or idiots) from lunatics for the purposes of property law. All social classes ostracised those with obvious mental disorder but otherwise society seems to have more or less ignored such people until around the 18th century. A reluctance to interfere with the divinely ordained nature of society, combined with the ability of an agricultural economy to contain a certain amount of mental disorder may have accounted for this lack of interest and concern. But for various reasons around the middle of the eighteenth century a movement grew to build hospitals and asylums to care for, or at least confine, lunatics. (These asylums were intended for the mentally ill, but since there was little or no separate provision many mentally handicapped people were confined in them.) This movement can be ascribed to a number of causes; the onset of the industrial revolution, with the technical skills which it demanded of workers and the shift from the country to the town which it created, probably brought to light the existence of a sizeable body of people who could not look after themselves. The asylum movement was an honourable attempt to remove mentally handicapped people from inappropriate confinement in prisons and workhouses and from the "trade in lunacy" (ie private housing in which lunatics were confined) which Lord Shaftesbury fought against. Asylums were intended to provide a more humane form of care. Within a hundred years came the recognition that among those who were classed as lunatics there was a discrete group of people who were not ill but "mentally defective" or "feeble minded". The concept of mental handicap thus started life as a variant of mental illness and despite later attempts to define it as a social problem the link with medicine – albeit as a poor relation of general medicine – was established. Apart from some early attempts to found schools for mentally handicapped children, public provision followed the pattern set by mental illness with the building of larger and larger asylums.

11

As happened so often in the field of lunacy reform the early efforts of enlightened philanthropists in providing "schools" gave way to the building of remote prison-like establishments to which the outcasts of the Victorian moral code could be consigned.

21. By the end of the nineteenth century the rise of the Eugenics Movement led to fears that the national intelligence would be lowered if the "feeble minded" were allowed to propagate freely. Sterilisation or at least segregation from the community seemed the only answer. Despite this generally gloomy picture, by the beginning of the twentieth century various voluntary organisations were attempting to revive the early educational and caring approach, by establishing training courses for mental health workers and training and occupation centres for mentally handicapped people. The 1913 Mental Deficiency Acts had recognised the problem as primarily a social rather than a medical phenomenon but care in the community with appropriate supervision was still regarded by the majority of the experts as second best to the "specialised" hospital or asylum environment. Nevertheless the 1913 Acts did establish the principle of providing training and occupation for mentally handicapped people even if local authorities were slow in establishing day centres for this purpose. Gradually through the 1920s and 30s the emphasis shifted from containment to active care and by the outbreak of the second world war such features as open wards, community care, mental health social workers, special schools and occupation and training centres were all regarded as appropriate components of the mental handicap picture. Sadly the staff and accommodation shortages imposed by the war meant "the return of the locked door, of inactivity, of isolation".[8]

Patterns of Nursing and Care

22. With the pressure towards specialised care for people with mental handicap came the organisation and professionalisation of the carers. In the mid-19th century the only staff training was that which some asylums conducted for themselves. In 1885 the Royal Medico-Psychological Association published a handbook of instruction for nursing the insane and 5 years later established a 2 year training course with a final examination and certificate. Within nine years over 100 asylums were participating in the scheme and 500–600 certificates were being granted each year. By the end of the century the staff giving direct care were thus able to obtain some kind of nurse training. In 1919 two General Nursing Councils (for England and Wales and for Scotland) were established by Acts of Parliament, and two Registers of nurses were established. After a "period of grace", during which existing nurses could Register by virtue of experience, Registration was limited to those who had completed the recognised training. The two Registers were divided into parts – for general, SRN (RGN in Scotland); sick children's, RSCN; fever, RFN; mental, RMN; and mental subnormality, RNMD (later changed to RNMS in England) nurses. Disagreements between the GNCs and the RMPA meant that for 25 years both organisations awarded their own certificates in mental handicap nursing, although the RMPA attracted far more entrants. The RMPA claimed that the GNCs' syllabuses were inappropriate to mental handicap and the theoretical examinations were too rigorous, while the GNCs wished to ensure uniformity across the different parts of the Register. When

12

the NHS came into being in 1948 over half of the 6,500 (whole time equivalent) nurses working in mental handicap hospitals in England and Wales were either qualified or in training for the RMPA or GNC qualifications; (the majority of these held or were training for the RMPA certificate).

23.   Although nurses played the main rôle in the care of mentally handicapped people, teachers and social workers were also involved. On the teaching side, the work of Itard in early 19th Century France, and later of Seguin, had engendered a belief that mentally handicapped people could be "socialised" by humane treatment. Thus the early "mental deficiency institutions" were "schools" in which it was hoped to train these people to be, or at least to appear normal. The first public educational institutions for mentally handicapped people were the Darenth Training Schools established in 1870 by the Metropolitan Asylums Board. Pressure from voluntary bodies and the example of the London School Board's special schools led to the passing of the Elementary Education (Defective and Epileptic Children) Act in 1899. This Act empowered (but did not require) local authorities to provide special schools or classes for "mentally deficient" children up to the age of 16. A further Act in 1914 made the powers of the 1899 Act compulsory and the Education Act of 1921 gave local authorities the duty of educating educable mentally handicapped children, leaving the ineducable to the Mental Deficiency Authorities. But by 1929 of the 33,000 ascertained mentally handicapped children in England and Wales (ie those known to the authorities) less than half were attending day special schools with under 3 per cent in residential accommodation. Added to this it was believed that there were about 18,000 unascertained mentally handicapped children. Although this legislation laid the foundation for special education it was left to the voluntary organisations to provide training for the special teachers. As in other areas the second world war prevented advances being made just at the time when opinion was ready for a dynamic approach to the care of mentally handicapped people. By 1948 the need for education and training was recognised by the experts but not fully met by the local authorities.

24.   The rôle of social workers in the field of mental handicap could be said to have grown out of the activities of the voluntary organisations. The services provided under the 1913 Mental Deficiency Act led to the development of a body of local authority and voluntary staff experienced in the training, occupation and supervision of mentally handicapped people. Mental health workers, however, tended to view mental handicap as a static medical condition and to assume that people living in institutions must automatically be more severely handicapped than those living in the community. This meant that there were, initially, a lack of active rehabilitative programmes in mental handicap. On the other hand the supervision of "ascertained defectives" under the 1913 Act led to the growth of "a helpful counselling service to parents of handicapped children, and provided the knowledge which led to the establishment of facilities for training in the community".[9] It was with mentally handicapped people and their families that untrained social workers began to develop community casework as a method of practice. The Central Association for Mental Welfare ran courses for serving mental health workers during the inter-war years and, by the work which they did during the second world war, social workers established themselves as a necessary element of the mental health scene. By 1948 the principle of local authority provision of mental

13

handicap services was accepted but, like all other services, insufficiently developed.

The NHS—and After

25. According to the Royal Commission on the Law Relating to Mental Illness and Mental Deficiency (1954–1957)[10] one of the aims of the 1944–1948 welfare state legislation was to distinguish between the social welfare functions and the hospital functions of the old Public Assistance institutions, and to divide these functions between the new local authority welfare service and hospital service accordingly. But this policy was not adopted for the mental health services and all mental deficiency institutions, of both hospital and welfare type, were transferred to the NHS hospital authorities. With hindsight it seems strange that this fateful decision appears to have been so sparsely documented. There were however a number of factors which may have influenced the decision. Firstly, it must be remembered that at this time mental handicap services were part of the wider mental health services and because of the smaller numbers involved mental handicap inevitably took second place to mental illness. In the 1940's the idea was current that conditions of the mind and body should be considered together, and the psychiatrists looked to many of the traditions and patterns of the general medical services as a model for the mental health services. A separate mental health service would, to many of those involved, have implied a second class service. Similarly the medical superintendents in the mental handicap hospitals would not have wanted to be treated differently from their colleagues in the mental illness hospitals. But the overriding factor in placing mental handicap within the health service was, in all probability, time. The politicans acknowledged that the mental health legislation was a complicated field in need of review. The White Paper "A National Health Service"[11] referred to the difficulty presented by the inclusion of the mental health service in the NHS, a difficulty which would remain until "a full restatement of the law of lunacy and mental deficiency can be undertaken. Yet, despite this difficulty, the mental health services should be included. The aim must be to reduce the distinctions drawn between mental ill-health and physical ill-health." Perhaps the politicans did not realise that they would have to wait 13 years for the results of that "restatement of the law". In the meantime, after 100 years in which educators, philanthropists, doctors and social workers had all tried to deal with the problem, the care of mentally handicapped people in residential accommodation was handed over to the health professions. Local authorities did however retain some interest in that they were responsible for after-care and day care facilities for mentally handicapped people.

26. Six years later, in 1954, the Royal Commission was established and the question of where and how mentally handicapped people should be cared for was once more a subject for debate. Kathleen Jones writes of the "three revolutions – pharmacological, administrative and legal" which commentators later regarded as having begun in the winter of 1953–4. Although the focus of these three changes was on mental illness, the link in the public mind between mental illness and mental handicap meant that changing attitudes in one sphere had considerable impact on the other. The "pharmacological revolution" was the development of the psychotropic drugs (or tranquillisers). The "administrative revolution", which was both facilitated and complemented by the new

14

drugs, involved the gradual shift towards the open ward, out-patient and short-term treatment, rehabilitation (with industrial therapy rather than containment in idleness), and the introduction of group therapy and patient participation. Finally, the "legal revolution" was the 1959 and 1960 Mental Health Acts which embodied some of these changes in a comprehensive new law covering both mentally ill and mentally handicapped people. While the Commission was sitting, in 1955, a White Paper containing proposals for amendment of the law on mental health was published in Scotland; further action was deferred pending the report of the Royal Commission.

27. The 1959/1960 Acts were the climax to the work of the Royal Commission. The Commission's terms of reference were limited to legal and administrative considerations, with the emphasis on the legal machinery for certifying patients as mentally ill or subnormal. But, as had happened in the past, public concern about wrongful detention led to a re-appraisal of the mental health services as a whole and to recommendations for improvement. The Commission was sitting at a time when there was renewed interest in the problems of mentally disordered people and its report both endorsed and gave an impetus to the move towards community care – "There should be a general re-orientation away from institutional care in its present form and towards community care" (Recommendation 4, Part V). It is difficult to chart the progress of the ideas about mental handicap which were current in the 1950's and 1960's, but the work of particular individuals and institutions seems to have had a considerable influence in shaping informed opinion. Certainly the report of the Royal Commission was a positive landmark on the road to community care, and signified the beginning of the end of the belief that large mental handicap hospitals were the best place for severely mentally handicapped people – "It is not now generally considered in the best interests of patients who are fit to live in the general community that they should live for long periods in large or remote institutions such as the present mental and mental deficiency hospitals, in which they are inevitably largely cut off from the normal world and from mixing with other people". (Para 601).

The Development of Mental Handicap Nursing 1948–1978

28. The changing attitudes of the post war years were reflected in the activities of the nursing profession which was beginning to accept the need for a new orientation in training for psychiatric nurses. The advent of the NHS proved the spur to ending the disagreement about examinations between the RMPA and the GNCs; it was agreed that after 1951 no further candidates would be admitted to the RMPA exams and existing certificate holders would be registered as qualified whether or not they transferred to the GNC Registers (as RMN or RNMS). In Scotland holders of the RMPA certificate were granted Registration as RNMD, through a concession in 1948–1952; thereafter entrance to the Register was by examination only. In 1949 the GNC for England and Wales conducted a survey[12] which showed that mental handicap hospitals had difficulty in recruiting staff. Although 48 of the 53 mental deficiency colonies and hospitals in operation had nurses in training (mostly for the RMPA certificate rather than the Register) many of the trainees were people who had not been accepted for general nurse training. The survey concluded that there was a great need for an appropriate mental handicap nurse training.

15

29. In 1951 the General Nursing Councils were reconstituted and two statutory Mentl Nurses Committees were established. When the new Councils came into being mental handicap nurses in England and Wales accounted for less than 500 names on a total Register of over 140,000 (although the RMPA had issued a large number (4,700) of certificates in mental handicap nursing over the past 80 years). The main problems confronting the new Mental Nurses Committees were to introduce: (a) appropriate entry requirements and (b) a more relevant syllabus for mental handicap nurse training. A major obstacle to progress in either field was the lack of a real alternative to the Register for mental handicap nurses. The Rolls of nurses, which had been introduced in 1944 to provide a different training for nurses in the practical situation working under the supervision of Registered nurses, were, unlike the Registers, not divided into parts. Although in theory any hospital which could meet the necessary conditions could become approved for training for the Roll the majority of mental handicap hospitals could not provide for the required general nursing component. Even for the Register the training provided for the mental handicap part was biased towards general nursing and the Preliminary Examination, which was common to all parts of the Register, required experience which it was difficult to obtain in mental handicap hospitals. There was thus no specific training in the nursing of people with mental handicap for the Roll, and an inappropriately general bias in training for the Register. In 1957 the Mental Nurses Committee of England and Wales recommended a new syllabus for the RNMS qualification which was more closely related to the needs of mental handicap nurses. The common preliminary examination was thus replaced by a specific intermediate examination for mental handicap student nurses. Similar changes were made in Scotland in 1964.

30. Progress on minimum educational entry standards hinged on the widening of the Roll to include mental handicap nurses. It was the lack of minimum entry standards which many regarded as the reason for the high wastage rate in student nurse training, but the Minister of Health was not prepared to see minimum educational standards until there was an assured route into mental handicap nursing for the academically less able, so that recruitment should not be affected. Eventually in 1964 legislation was passed to establish training for the Roll for psychiatric nurses in England and Wales and to allow psychiatric nursing assistants to enrol by virtue of experience; 16,000 nurses did so as State Enrolled Mental Nurses SEN(M) or State Enrolled Mental Subnormality Nurses SEN(MS). The way was thus clear for an educational standard of entry and when this was introduced in 1966 the expected increase in applicants and drop in the wastage rate occurred. The Roll in Scotland has not been divided into parts.

31. Having established a two-tier structure for mental handicap nursing efforts have been made by the profession over the last 10-15 years to improve patient care and nurse training in line with changing attitudes to the care of mentally handicapped people. Major changes were made in the syllabus for Registered nurses in 1957 (1964 in Scotland) in response to pressure from mental handicap nurses in the field. The most recent changes in the syllabus (in 1970 in England and Wales and 1972 in Scotland) reflect the increasing emphasis on community care and recommend placements outside the hospital

16

in a variety of Local Authority departments. In 1972 the (Briggs) Committee on Nursing recommended that "A new caring profession for the mentally handicapped should emerge gradually. In the meantime, in the training of nurses in the field of mental handicap, increased emphasis should be placed on the social aspects of care". (REC. 74) This proposal was the logical result of the changing attitudes to mentally handicapped people and of the belief that the majority of patients did not need hospital care but rather "home" care, either in or out of hospital. A new curriculum for student (ie pre-Registration) nurses, including mental handicap nurses has recently been circulated for comment in Scotland. The proposed curriculum incorporates recommendations made by the Briggs Committee and in the Scottish White Paper (The Way Ahead).[13]

Local Authority Services 1948–1978

32. While the nursing profession was coming to accept the need to match nurse training to the newly recognised needs of mentally handicapped hospital patients there was a growing recognition that more local authority services were needed. The (Younghusband) Working Party on Social Workers in the Local Authority Health and Welfare Services (which reported in 1959)[14], assumed that "a considerable expansion and development of the local authority mental health service must be expected". (Para 38). Although the working party was primarily concerned with field social workers its report noted that "what is abundantly clear is that a considerable residential service [for the mentally ill and handicapped] will be required. It should be staffed by officers with a real understanding of the needs of the mentally disordered, and supported by a well developed community care service". (Para 455). By 1968 when the Seebohm Committee (On Local Authority and Allied Personal Social Services) reported, local authorities were providing, directly or indirectly (eg by using facilities provided by other local authorities or by voluntary organisations) the following specialist facilities: mental health social workers, day special schools, hostels for mentally handicapped people, boarding special schools, junior and adult training centres, and workshops and social centres for mentally disordered people. Residential accommodation was provided by local authorities as a welfare function (under Part III of the National Assistance Act) and by local health authorities (under the Mental Health Acts). In fact about 60 per cent of these (non-hospital) residential places were for elderly mentally handicapped people, so that the principle of providing life-time hostel accommodation for young amd middle aged mentally handicapped people had not yet been established. The Seebohm Committee took the view that services for mentally handicapped people suffered from duplication and lack of team work. The belief that services for mentally handicapped people should be as near normal as possible was gaining popularity and the Committee recommended that Junior Training Centres should be the responsibility of the local education authorities (where they were to be called special schools) who had the relevant expertise, while Adult Training Centres should be run by the proposed new social services, or social work departments.

Training in the Social Services

33. While the nursing profession was developing nurse training to meet the demands of different groups of patients the personal social services were also developing staff training courses. The large voluntary organisations led

the way in training for residential care but in 1947 the first statutory residential care training was introduced: the Central Training Council in Child Care (CTC) introduced 14 month courses for housemothers. These courses laid the foundations for the later Certificate in the Residential Care of Children and Young People. In 1967, following the recommendations of the Williams Committee, a generic two-year course for workers in children's homes and homes for elderly and handicapped people was introduced. On the field work side psychiatric social work was one of the first disciplines to acquire a recognised training with the introduction of the Association for Psychiatric Social Workers' Course in 1930. Other disciplines followed suit and the Council for Training in Social Work (CTSW) was established in 1962. In 1968 the CTSW extended its remit to residential social work and in 1969 it launched the first one year qualifying courses for senior staff in homes for elderly and handicapped people. These courses led to the award of the Certificate in Residential Social Work (CRSW).

34.   In October 1971 the Central Council for Education and Training in Social Work (CCETSW) was established to unify the existing councils. The following year CCETSW established a working party to consider education for residential social work; the future of the residential training courses and of CCETSW's own Certificate of Qualification in Social Work is considered in Chapter 5. In addition to fieldworkers and residential staff CCETSW acquired responsibility in 1974 for the training of day care staff, including instructors and managers in Adult Training Centres. Training for the staff of day centres for mentally handicapped children and adults had been pioneered by the National Association for Mental Health (MIND) and developed by the Training Council for Teachers of the Mentally Handicapped (TCTMH) which was established in 1964. The TCTMH had promoted courses for instructors/teachers and managers in both Junior and Adult Training Centres until 1971 when the JTCs were transferred to local education authorities as special schools. Thereafter teachers of mentally handicapped children were trained within mainstream teacher education. After the TCTMH handed over its responsibilities to CCETSW in 1974 the Diploma in the Training and Further Education of Mentally Handicapped Adults (Dip. TMHA) courses continued. Meanwhile CCETSW was considering the training needs of various groups of staff (other than social workers) in the field, residential, day, domiciliary and community services. The result of CCETSW's deliberations was the creation in 1975 of the Certificate in Social Service, a modular training scheme flexible enough to meet a wide range of needs. The Dip. TMHA courses are now being absorbed into the new CSS schemes.

A Decade of Plans and Enquiries 1959 – 1971

35.   The 1960's saw a slow, steady, essential, but nonetheless one-sided attempt to improve physical conditions in the mental handicap hospitals. It seemed that the momentum created by the report of the 1957 Royal Commission was not to be dissipated in the way of so many previous efforts at reform, but the emphasis was on "hardware" rather than "care". The Hospital Plan of 1962[16] and the Community Care Plan of 1963[17] reflected the new emphasis on community services. The Hospital Plan admittedly struck a warning note by emphasising that hospital services for mentally handicapped people could not be run down in the way that was envisaged for the mental illness

18

hospitals, but nevertheless community services – training centres, workshops, homes – were planned to complement the long-stay hospitals which would be needed for the foreseeable future. Sadly these plans proved to be over optimistic and escalating costs combined with recruitment difficulties meant that improvements were slow to materialise. A 1965 Ministry of Health circular[18] made suggestions for improving the effectiveness of the hospital services, stressing the need for joint planning by hospital and local authorities and re-emphasising the new attitude to patients which the Royal Commission Report required. Although the recommendations were mainly not specific or detailed, hospital authorities were asked to make the necessary improvements.

36.   This gentle pace of change was dramatically accelerated when in 1967 a newspaper published allegations of cruelty and malpractice at Ely Hospital, Cardiff. The Report of the Ely Committee of Inquiry[19] which was published in 1969, and others which followed in subsequent years, drew the attention of both the public and the government to the grave problems facing long-stay hospitals, including their lack of resources. New concepts in mental handicap care were being discussed by the theorists but strategies for disseminating the ideas to hospitals were lacking and the resources to implement them were in any case not available. The Ely Report, by stimulating public interest in mental handicap, precipitated both a new flow of funds and a re-allocation of resources to mental handicap hospitals to enable these ideas to be put into effect. Another result of the malpractice enquiries was the establishment in 1970 of the Hospital Advisory Service to provide an outside and independent check on the closed world of the long-stay hospital. This Service reported direct to the Secretary of State. In addition detailed practical measures to improve standards were drawn up and issued to Hospital Boards in 1969.[20] These were minimum standards to be achieved as rapidly as possible over the next few years with the help of a specific allocation of funds. They were only interim measures, however, because the general policy on mental handicap was already under discussion with a view to producing a major new policy statement. In the meantime hospitals were exhorted to improve staff/patient ratios, increase living and sleeping space, introduce routine ward level inter-disciplinary meetings and staff training schemes and increase the numbers of domestic staff. These recommendations were re-emphasised in a further communication in 1970. In the same year the Education (Handicapped Children) Act was passed and as from April 1971 the responsibility for educating all mentally handicapped children passed to the local education authorities. The Education (Scotland) (Mentally Handicapped Children) Act 1974 achieved the same result in Scotland. Once again the importance of providing the normal services available to other adults and children, or a near equivalent to normal services, was being recognised.

A New Policy Statement – 1971

37.   In 1971 the expected policy statement was issued in the form of a White Paper – "Better Services for the Mentally Handicapped". The policies outlined in the paper were a direct development from the proposals of the Royal Commission of 1957 but with specific targets (involving a shift in emphasis from hospital to community care to be achieved in the next 15–20 years) set for local and hospital authorities. Hospital authorities were asked

to improve existing facilities (continuing the measures begun in 1969) and to provide any new hospital places required in small or medium sized units of not more than 100–200 beds sited in the district they were to serve; local authorities were asked to continue to establish new Adult Training Centres and other day and family support services, but also to expand the provision of residential care. Regional Hospital Boards were asked to prepare plans, in conjunction with local authorities, for putting these policies into effect. But the task proved more difficult than had been expected and the onset of the local authority and NHS re-organisations meant that this exercise in co-operation had to be replaced by a new form of joint planning which is still in the process of development. Nevertheless the White Paper did lay down, for the first time, the basic principles on which services for the mentally handicapped should build. These principles emphasised that mentally handicapped people have the same needs and rights as other people and that where special services have to be provided these should be as much like normal social and public services and facilities as possible.

Recent History 1971 – 1978

38.   Achievements since 1971 were reviewed by the Secretary of State for Social Services in a speech to the National Society for Mentally Handicapped Children in February 1975. Inevitably there had been some disappointments to place alongside the undoubted progress which had been made; the two main areas of concern were the slow progress in providing local authority homes and the continuing survival of old fashioned attitudes towards mentally handicapped people. The first of these problems was a question of funds and there was some hope of improvement; the second problem was more complex. In her speech the Secretary of State announced that a National Development Group (NDG) for the Mentally Handicapped was to be established to advise Ministers on the development of policy. Since then the Group has produced five free pamphlets giving advice on various aspects of mental handicap services. These pamphlets have been well received by authorities and by those directly involved in care. The fact that 54,000 copies of Pamphlet 5 alone have been printed is an indication of the Group's success at provoking interest in new ideas for the delivery of mental handicap services. In the Spring of 1977 the Secretary of State asked the Group for their advice on a major problem – how to improve services in mental handicap hospitals within existing resources. Their report – "Helping Mentally Handicapped People in Hospital"[21] was published recently. Another body, the Development Team for the Mentally Handicapped, was also established in 1975. The Team was set up to give advice and assistance to the NHS and local social services departments in the planning and operation of services for mentally handicapped people and their families. Both the NDG and the Team are independent of the DHSS.

39.   The two new advisory bodies were intended to promote a wider dissemination of new ideas about mental handicap, but the questions of who should care for mentally handicapped people and how the residential care staff should acquire the knowledge and skills which the experts now thought necessary, required further examination. The Briggs Committee on Nursing (which reported in 1972) recommended radical changes in the training

of nurses. In particular the Committee recommended that "a new caring profession" for the mentally handicapped should emerge gradually. The Briggs modular nurse training, with its emphasis on common elements rather than particular skills, went against the trend of mental handicap nursing which was becoming more and more specialised, and the idea of a new caring profession caused concern among many mental handicap nurses. It was in this atmosphere of anxiety and uncertainty that our Committee was established in 1975. The most recent development in the field of mental handicap has been the publication of the White Paper on the Mental Health Act[22] which occurred too late for us to consider any implications it might have for residential care.

Services and Staff

40.   In para 3 we explained that we were unable to divorce staffing considerations from the structure within which care is delivered. Mental handicap residential institutions are for the most part located in the health service, since the development of local authority homes on any appreciable scale has taken place only recently. The majority of the staff caring for mentally handicapped people are therefore nurses, whose ethos derives from the nursing and medical world. One would expect mental handicap student and pupil nurses to look to other nurses, rather than to residential care staff in local authority homes for mentally handicapped people, for their peer group. For although the two groups of staff may be doing similar jobs their training, conditions of work, organisational hierarchy, career structure, and employing authority are different; such differences have an important effect on what is being taught. A "nurse" who is being taught in a "hospital" is bound to receive a different slant to her training from a "residential social worker/houseparent" who is working in a "hostel/home", even if both types of staff are taught the same subjects. These variables also colour the way in which what is learned in training is put into effect. Our terms of reference required us to focus on the job to be done and how people should be trained to do it, but to carry out our task we had to place training in the context of the services which are available now, or may be available in the future.

41.   We were asked to accept as our starting point the pattern of services recommended in the 1971 White Paper. Briefly these were a shift in the balance from hospital to community care with a rapid expansion in local authority services, a relative reduction in the numbers cared for within the hospital service, and the development of a decentralised hospital service which would be able to link closely with local community services. The White Paper recommended that children should not be removed from their own neighbourhood for residential care except as a last resort. There was also the commitment to improve, but not to extend, the existing large hospitals. The White Paper figures suggested that an increase in local authority residential places of more than 600 per cent was required, alongside a drop of nearly 50 per cent in hospital places. Thus, even without our recommendations, services for mentally handicapped people are in a state of change. As the balance of services shifts, so too the staffing of the services will change, with many more staff being employed by social services departments and with better nurse/patient ratios in health authorities. Staff will therefore need to be trained to cope with a variety of surroundings. In addition to this the White Paper figures themselves may need to be amended in the light of experience. For

these reasons training will need to provide staff with a range of skills to be used flexibly as the content and location of their work varies over time. We also had to bear in mind that the implementation of the Briggs Report on nursing would also affect the way in which nurses in mental handicap hospitals would be trained.

THE SHAPE OF THE REPORT

From Principles to Practice

42. In this chapter we have set out the facts as we see them, as the background to our Enquiry. But we decided that to plan for the future we should go back to first principles and examine the needs (and rights) of mentally handicapped people. As a first step we examined the 613 pieces of written evidence, and the oral evidence submitted to us, plus the OPCS survey and the evidence gathered on our visits. Because this evidence provided us with an important insight into the views of staff and parents we have thought it right to include an analysis of the findings at an early stage in the report. Chapter 2 is therefore devoted to evidence. Having assembled the relevant data our next move was to draw up a list of fundamental principles concerning mentally handicapped people. These principles, which we set out in Chapter 3, provide the backbone to all our thinking about mental handicap. Around these principles we built a model of the way in which we believe care should be delivered. In this model, we describe the kinds of accommodation and the range of experiences which should be available to mentally handicapped people at different stages in their lives, and the philosophy behind the services to be delivered. In subsequent chapters we take up and develop the 3 main strands of our model; the number of residential care staff required, the training of residential care staff, and the organisational and management structures within which staff should be deployed. In the chapters dealing with these three themes we explain our objectives and describe the means by which we believe they can be achieved.

Normal Patterns of Life

43. The fundamental feature of our model is that mentally handicapped people should have access to general facilities and services, by which we mean everything from social work services and home helps to public transport and public swimming pools. Only where the mentally handicapped person needs something over and above the general provision, or where it is either impractical (eg because of physical disability) or undesirable for him to use general services should separate, specialist provisions be made. All of our recommendations flow from our belief in the primacy of a "normal" lifestyle for mentally handicapped people.

Manpower

44. In Chapter 4 we discuss the residential care staff manpower required to implement our model. We consider the difficulties of deciding on correct staff/resident ratios and test 2 possible means of estimating the residential care staff numbers required. Since it is clear that a large increase is necessary we consider ways of building up staff numbers to the desired level.

Training of Residential Care Staff

45.   Our training model is intended to produce residential care staff who can create the normal lifestyle to which mentally handicapped people have a right. Chapter 5 sets out the qualities we think staff who will care for mentally handicapped people require, and describes the training model which we have formulated to meet these needs. In this, as in all other aspects of our work, we started from the principle of looking at mentally handicapped people first and foremost as people. We observed how all people in residential care had certain needs in common and certain special needs and we devised a staff training programme to reflect this union of generic and specialist elements.

Organisation and Management

46.   Our views on the organisation of staff working in mental handicap residential care are given in Chapter 6. Our organisational model is one of teamwork, in which staff with varying degrees of training and experience work together without rigid demarcations. Within the team we distinguished various levels of work (Basic – Trainee – Qualified – Advanced) which are required in direct residential care (ie at unit level). We also consider the organisation of residential care staff at higher management and policy making levels. The structure we propose would operate in both health and social services authorities.

Finance and Conclusions

47.   The final two chapters of our report are devoted to the financial implications of our recommendations, with our own suggestions on priorities (Chapter 7), and to a summary of our conclusions (Chapter 8).

Supplementary Information

48.   We have included three appendices in our report, in addition to the separate volume containing our OPCS survey. Appendix A is the question-naire which we supplied to all those who submitted written evidence; Appendix B gives the list of those who submitted written and/or oral evidence and Appendix C lists the places we visited.

CHAPTER 2 – EVIDENCE

SOURCES

49.   In considering the task set before us we did not wish to rely solely on our own collective experience; we wanted to hear from all those with an interest in mental handicap and we hoped to build up a picture of the views of nursing and residential care staff. We therefore gathered evidence in four ways: by seeking written and oral evidence, by commissioning a survey and by making visits.

Written Evidence

50.   We were anxious that all members of staff working in the field of mental handicap, parents and friends of mentally handicapped people and everyone else with an interest, should be aware of our existence and purpose and should be encouraged to submit evidence, either individually or collectively. We therefore invited written evidence from persons and organisations prominent in the field of mental handicap, and from members of the general public. We did this by writing direct to the relevant organisations and by sending a press notice to a large number of newspapers and journals. A questionnaire based on our terms of reference, with a cover note from the Chairman, was supplied to every person or group accepting the invitation to submit a personal or professional opinion on the care of mentally handicapped people. Since we were particularly concerned to have the views of nursing and local authority residential care staff about their work we asked health and social services authorities to publicise our invitation to submit evidence and our questionnaire in all mental handicap hospitals and residential establishments. The questionnaire was designed by a group of Committee members and comprised 15 questions (see Appendix A), the main purpose of which was to structure replies so that an analysis could be carried out at a later date. Those who did not wish to use the questionnaire were encouraged to submit evidence as they wished.

Oral Evidence

51.   It was clear to us that we needed to supplement the written evidence with oral evidence. All those who requested an opportunity to discuss their written evidence with us or who preferred to give oral evidence were given the opportunity to come and talk to us. We also invited representatives of professional and statutory bodies to give oral evidence and to discuss with us matters relating to our brief.

Survey

52.   We asked the Social Survey Division of the Office of Population Censuses and Surveys to carry out a survey of nursing staff in mental handicap hospitals and residential care staff in local authority homes for mentally handicapped people. This survey was intended to provide information about the present rôle of the nursing and local authority residential care staff and about *their* views on some issues relating to their possible future rôles. (The full survey is published separately as Volume II of this report.)

Visits

53.   The fourth aspect of evidence gathering was undertaken by Committee members visiting hospitals, homes and Adult Training Centres (ATCs)

scattered throughout England, Scotland and Wales. On these visits we discussed our remit with staff, individually or on a group basis, and sought the views of all who wished to talk to us.

54. *We are grateful to all those who gave written or oral evidence, took part in the survey, or demonstrated their expertise during the visits, for the important contribution which they have made to our thinking about the care of mentally handicapped people.*

WRITTEN EVIDENCE

55. Altogether, 613 pieces of written evidence were received, ranging from single page letters to long and closely argued papers. Many of the submissions presented by organisations have been published. We were particularly pleased to receive much written evidence from staff who had organised working parties and discussion groups before submitting written evidence as a group.

Analysis

56. We recognised that an analysis of the written evidence which consisted of completed questionnaires, partially completed questionnaires, reports or research projects would be difficult if not impossible. The first analysis of all the written evidence was undertaken by nominated members of the Committee who looked at written evidence by grouping it into four main staff groups, ie nursing; local authority; doctors/psychologists/remedial professions; and voluntary/independent. A further independent analysis was undertaken by a postgraduate student at Birmingham University under the supervision of a member of our Committee. Figure 6 below, taken from this independent study, shows the professional identity of those who submitted written evidence to us.

FIGURE 6 – ANALYSIS OF THE PROFESSIONAL IDENTITY OF THE RESPONDENTS

Professional group	No.	%
Nurses	220	35
(Of these, 22% (137) are single respondents, and 13% (83) are group respondents. 2% (10) of the total nurses are community-based.)		
Nursing tutors	26	4
Nursing and midwifery committees	21	3
Community Health Councils	19	3
General practitioners	2	0.5
Psychologists (clinical)	16	3
Paediatricians	5	1
Psychiatrists (consultant)	20	3
Remedial professions	22	3
Health authorities: groups and single employees	63	10
Trades Unions	4	1
Professional associations	45	7
Independent multi-disciplinary groups	2	0.5
Independent research contributors	7	1
Voluntary workers	3	0.5
Families	17	3
Charities	23	4
Unknown status	3	0.5
Education	10	2
Residential workers	19	3
Adult training centre staff	12	2
Social workers	11	2
Local authorities (SSD admin and exec)	43	7
Total	613	100

The percentages are given to the nearest 0.5%.
Source: Independent study.

25

The list gives the number of contributions; certain groups have submitted more than one piece of evidence such as, for example, two divisions of the Royal College of Psychiatrists.

57. As expected, the biggest response to our request for written evidence came from nursing staff in mental handicap hospitals (35 per cent). Nurses' opinions were also, of course, represented by nursing and midwifery committees, by nurse tutors, and in the mixed groups making up some of the health authority contributions. 21 responses (3 per cent) were received from individual psychiatrists. The medical profession was, however, well represented in terms of professional associations. The response from residential workers, social workers and ATC staff was less than might have been expected, ie 2 per cent in each case. Of groups submitting written evidence 73 per cent were groups of National Health Service respondents, 17.5 per cent of local authority respondents and 9.5 per cent of independent respondents.

Services

58. In respect of priorities for services the most frequent proposal (37 per cent of replies) was for more residential units outside hospitals; 35 per cent asked for more education and work facilities and for more day care resources; and 35 per cent asked for more information and casework support for families. The other significant group of 27 per cent requested more domiciliary support for families. The smallest group of replies was the 6 per cent in favour of keeping large hospitals.

Tasks and Rôles

59. The evidence suggested that the mental handicap nurse is perceived as more actively caring by her nursing colleagues than by field workers from local authorities. The latter seem to attribute to the nurse a more passive "looking-after" rôle. The general view of the nurse did, however, depict her as helping to habilitate her mentally handicapped patients. The evidence suggested that inter-disciplinary responsibility is generally acceptable to staff and others. There was very little support for the concept of overall clinical responsibility for the doctor. Lack of co-operation and lack of specialist staff were commented on vociferously by respondents from both health and social services authorities.

Manpower

60. The concept of "common core" training (ie common to health, social services and teaching staff) was highly rated and supported by health authorities, nursing tutors, professional (medical) associations and nurses. The nurses were anxious about the lack of refresher and re-orientation courses; the lower ranking nurses were particularly concerned about opportunities for retraining and the chance to supplement the training they had already received.

Organisation of Services

61. The most popular proposal (27 per cent of replies) for re-organising services was the idea of a co-ordinated service jointly planned by NHS, social services and education authorities. All the major staff groups gave significant votes for this idea. There was a low vote for the idea of a new centrally-funded

specialist service. The suggestion that mental handicap hospitals should eventually be phased out received poor support (6 per cent) in general, although a significant proportion of the charities and the health authorities voted for this option.

Summary

62.   Our own analysis of the written evidence indicated that:

(a) There was substantial support for the 1971 White Paper policies;

(b) There was a strong preference for inter-disciplinary rather than medical/clinical responsibility;

(c) There was strong support for small group living;

(d) The present staff training schemes constrain or prevent individual effectiveness in meeting the tasks related to mental handicap;

(e) Nurses are expected to make important decisions but their formal authority is not recognised;

(f) No person, however well trained, can apply their knowledge to the care of mentally handicapped people without specialist training in mental handicap;

(g) Staff training schemes for residential care workers should include a large mental handicap component;

(h) The severely mentally handicapped person's needs must be catered for in any future training programme;

(i) There are doubts as to whether the "mainstream" Briggs proposals would be able to provide adequate training for staff giving residential care to mentally handicapped people;

(j) Formal training should be provided for unqualified staff, eg nursing assistants.

ORAL EVIDENCE

63.   We took oral evidence on 37 occasions, mostly through an appointed Sub-Committee but on occasions in full Committee. In the main the oral evidence followed the lines of the written evidence, ie support for the White Paper; some dissatisfaction with present nurse training schemes; a belief that the present CSS training schemes are too generic; support for small group living; a need for more staff; plus various suggestions for improving the organisation of services.

64.   The meetings with the statutory bodies, professional organisations and unions proved most informative and aided us considerably in our work.

27

SURVEY

65.   We commissioned the Social Survey Division of the Office of Population Censuses and Surveys (OPCS) to conduct for us a survey of nurses and local authority residential staff caring for mentally handicapped people. This survey is published as Volume II of our report. In paragraphs 66–81 below we have reproduced the introductory summary to the survey.

Aim of the Survey

66.   *The intention of the survey was to provide information from a representative sample of nursing and residential home staff on their present and future roles, training and career structures. A principal objective was to find what emphasis staff placed on the social aspects of caring, that is on developing their residents' individual abilities and enabling them to live as independently as possible. Interviews were carried out with 967 nurses from 56 mental handicap hospitals and with 390 residential care staff from 103 local authority homes. In addition, information was obtained on the present abilities of the residents and staff ratios within a representative sample of (297) wards in these hospitals and within all the homes. Almost all of the hospitals and homes which were approached agreed to take part in the survey and interviews were conducted with about 95 per cent of the selected individuals.*

Summary of the Survey's Findings

Characteristics of the Staff

67.   *Although the majority of the staff were women (70 per cent of the nurses and 82 per cent of the home staff) almost half or more of the staff in the more senior grades were men. Half of the nursing and care assistants, but less than a tenth of the more senior staff, worked part-time; the part-time staff mainly being married women. About a quarter of the staff had obtained at least one "A" level or 5 "O" levels but almost two thirds had no "O" levels (or equivalent qualifications). Very few of the nurses had ever worked in a mental handicap home but 40 per cent of the home staff had previously been nurses, including 20 per cent with experience of mental handicap. About three quarters of the nurses in each of the trained nursing grades were qualified in mental handicap nursing; the remainder were qualified in general or psychiatric nursing. Most of the officers in charge of the homes were qualified either in nursing or in social work (or both in a few cases) but a third of them held no formal qualifications. 27 per cent of all the nurses were born outside the United Kingdom and about half of these nurses had come from a developing country. However, a much higher proportion than this of the trainee nurses and of the younger trained nurses were born in developing countries, (about 30 per cent). Only a tenth of the home staff were born outside the UK and most of these had come from Eire.*

The Wards and Homes and their Residents

68.   *90 per cent of the wards and 75 per cent of the homes were for adults and these were classified into four ability groups:–*

(a)   *High ability (36 per cent of the adult wards) – with residents who generally seemed to be able to look after themselves with a minimum of supervision;*

(b)   *Average ability (34 per cent of the adult wards) – most of these*

28

residents were considered to need some help with their basic care *(especially in washing or dressing)*;

(c) *Low ability (19 per cent of the adult wards)* – with residents who needed considerable assistance with their basic care and were often incontinent or considered to have a behaviour problem *(for example being aggressive)*;

(d) *Non-ambulant with very low ability (10 per cent of the adult wards)* – three-quarters of these residents could not walk by themselves and most of them needed assistance with feeding as well as in washing and dressing. Almost all the adult homes were in the high ability group. A much higher proportion of patients in the non-ambulant and children's wards, than in the other units, suffered from various physical handicaps or illnesses – in particular two thirds of the former suffered from cerebral palsy (spasticity).

69.   There was a lower average number of residents in the homes than in the wards and the homes had better staff ratios (calculated as the average number of residents whom each staff member was looking after during the daytime), particularly in comparison with the high ability adult wards. In the hospitals the staff ratios were related to the ability level of the patients in that there were fewer patients per nurse in the low ability and non-ambulant wards than in the others. Two factors which contributed to the homes having relatively better staff ratios than the hospitals were firstly that more of the home residents attended an occupational centre and secondly that the home staff worked more overtime.

The Work Carried Out by the Nursing and Care Staff

70.   The proportion of the staff who, on their last working day, had spent over an hour on one of four tasks which form part of their social caring role (teaching, playing with residents, going on outgoings or encouraging them to organise their own activities) was similar in the adult wards and homes (about 44 per cent), but rather lower in the children's wards (35 per cent) than in the children's homes (55 per cent). Nurses working with the lower ability patients or in wards with relatively poor staff ratios spent more time than staff in the other units on providing basic care for their patients. Conversely staff working with higher ability residents or in wards with relatively good staff ratios seemed to be able to place more emphasis on helping their residents to do tasks like feeding, washing and dressing themselves. According to the staff, behaviour modification programmes were used in a third of the wards and a fifth of the homes, the ward or home staff usually being involved in carrying out the programmes. The question of whether the nursing and care staff spend too much time on domestic and administrative work is discussed. Only a few of the staff expressed dissatisfaction with the domestic side of their work but a third of the more senior ward and home staff were dissatisfied with their administrative work.

The Way the Wards and Homes were Run

71.   In general fewer restrictions or routines were adopted in the homes than in the hospitals but there were only minor differences between the adult homes and the high ability wards. There appeared to be some scope for allowing the residents to live more independently in some of the homes and wards in each

29

ability group and particularly within a few wards which seemed to be run on traditional institutional lines. There was slightly more stability in the staffing of the homes than of the wards in that, for example, 80 per cent of the officers in charge of homes compared with 70 per cent of the ward sisters or charge nurses had worked in their unit for a year or longer.

72.   *Half of the nurses, but hardly any of the home staff, were obliged to wear uniforms. The wards in which the nurses wore uniforms tended to be run in a more institutional way than the other wards. The arrangements for and frequency of contacts with relatives and voluntary workers were similar in the hospitals and homes. During the previous week almost a fifth of the residents had been visited by relatives and voluntary workers had assisted in activities with the residents in about half of the units.*

Contact with Staff in Other Professions and Influence over Decisions on Individual Residents

73.   *Most, but not all, of the more senior ward and home staff had frequent discussions with staff from their residents' occupational centre or with the school teachers. However, about half of the more junior staff had never taken part in this type of discussion. The vast majority of the ward sisters/charge nurses, but only half of the officers in charge, had discussed the progress of at least one of their residents with a mental handicap consultant within the last six months. Conversely almost all of the officers in charge, but only two-thirds of the ward sisters/charge nurses had had this type of discussion with a social worker within the same period.*

74.   *Just over a third of the ward sisters and a fifth of the officers in charge said that case conferences were never held on their residents. Within the hospitals this seemed to be linked to many of the ward sisters and nursing officers feeling that their views were not fully taken into account in making decisions concerning their patients, for example with respect to admitting new patients or transferring them. The ward sisters who were rarely involved in making these decisions tended to have more limited objectives for their patients and to have a more pessimistic view of the scope for developing the potential abilities of mentally handicapped people.*

The Staff's General Attitudes Towards Mentally Handicapped People

75.   *In general both the nurses and the home staff seemed to appreciate the value of developing the individual potential of mentally handicapped people. The home staff were generally in favour of community provision and integration of mentally handicapped people whereas more of the nurses were sceptical about the quality of care at present provided for discharged patients who lived in homes. The staff's attitudes towards the questions of sterilisation and of whether to discourage or encourage sexual relationships amongst mentally handicapped people suggested that this was an area which presents them with difficulties. About 40 per cent of both groups of staff felt that more mentally handicapped patients or residents should be sterilised.*

30

The Staff's View of their Present Aims

76.   The staff's aims for their residents were related to some extent to the ability level of the residents. However, more of the staff from the adult homes, than from the high ability adult wards, considered that their most important aim was to enable their residents to live independently in society. About a quarter of the nurses in the lower ability wards felt that their main objective was to provide (rather than teach) basic care or to give medical attention. The senior nursing staff tended to have a more optimistic view than the ward nurses of the present aims for the hospital patients. The staff's aims and general attitudes towards mentally handicapped people did not appear to depend on whether their unit had a relatively good or poor staff ratio (after taking into account the ability levels of their residents).

The Staff's Views on their Work at Present and in the Future

77.   Of various tasks that they carried out at present almost half of the nurses and three-quarters of the home staff liked part of their social caring role the best. But an appreciable proportion of the nurses (22 per cent) most preferred their clinical nursing work. The majority of both staff groups felt that in the future they should place a greater emphasis on their social role either by helping their residents to develop to their full potential or by providing a more homelike, family atmosphere. About a third of the staff suggested that more community services or community care should be developed, including half of the nursing officers who thought that their nurses should give more domiciliary support or advice to parents.

The Staff's Views on their Relationship with Other Professional Staff

78.   At least half of the nursing and home staff would have preferred to have had more contact with staff in all but one of the professions covered by the survey. The exception was ward doctors or GPs with whom most of the staff felt they had sufficient contact at present. Two factors which were found to be related to dissatisfaction amongst the nursing or home staff with the present role or service provided by other professional staff were, firstly, a lack of influence over decisions on individual residents from their units and, secondly, a lack of regular discussions with the other professional staff (especially with respect to staff from the training centres and psychologists).

The Staff's Views on their Careers

79.   In many ways the careers of the nurses seemed to be more closely linked to providing social care for mentally handicapped people than to doing clinical nursing. Recently recruited nurses had mainly been attracted by the opportunity to do a caring job rather than by the opportunity to become, or continue to be, a nurse. Similarly most of the nurses thought they would still be working with mentally handicapped people in five years' time. Nevertheless, an appreciable proportion of the nurses had previously worked with other types of patients (41 per cent) or thought they would like to transfer to other types of nursing in the future (32 per cent). A lack of career opportunities for the enrolled nurses and nursing and care assistants seemed to lead to a relatively higher proportion

31

of these staff feeling that chances of promotion were inapplicable to them, or to dissatisfaction with their prospects.

Training in the Care of Mentally Handicapped People

80. It is questionable whether the nursing and care assistants or enrolled nurses receive sufficient training on the scope for developing the full potential of their residents. With respect to nursing or care assistants this seems to be related to a general lack of training for staff in their grades in that, for example, almost half of them said they had not received any training or advice on ways of dealing with behaviour problems. The enrolled nurses seemed to be more attached to their clinical nursing role than the registered nurses which may stem partly from their formal training placing undue emphasis on the clinical and medical aspects of their work. The changes in the syllabus for student nurses in 1970 appear to have led to recently trained nurses having a rather more optimistic view of the scope for developing their residents' abilities but, in practice, they do not seem to spend more time on teaching their patients or encouraging them to be more independent. Almost half of the senior nursing staff who expressed a view on this issue felt that the students' syllabus placed too much emphasis on clinical nursing.

81. There was no evidence to suggest that the type of care provided in the homes depended on whether or not the officers in charge had obtained a recognised training qualification, or on whether they were qualified in nursing or social work. About half of the home staff who had recently attended a social work course felt that the educational side of their work and the type of activities they could do with the residents had not been covered on their course.

VISITS

82. Members of the Committee visited 19 hospitals, 23 homes, 11 ATCs and 2 Certificate in Social Service courses in England, Scotland and Wales. During the visits opportunities were made available for staff to speak individually or in groups to individuals or groups of Committee members. We were most impressed with the concern of the staff about the effect which any new developments following our report might have on their patients/residents. We would like to express our appreciation to the staff of the hospitals, homes, ATCs and colleges we visited for their many kindnesses and their interest in our work.

83. One of the main concerns raised during these visits was the staff's own fears about their future if changes were to take place. Questions such as "What will happen to my present qualification?", "Will I lose my lead?" (salary allowance for psychiatric nurses), "Will I lose my Mental Health Officer status?", "What about my professional status?", etc were frequently voiced. On the other hand we were often told that any recommendations which would benefit mentally handicapped people and provide the staff with a better training and at least equal pay and conditions of service would be given fair condideration.

84. The visits we undertook not only enabled us to see a variety of mental handicap services and talk to the staff but also allowed us to identify with the

concerns of those who are most vulnerable—the residents and the staff. If we needed any further encouragement in the task before us it was during the visits that our commitment to the residents and to those caring for them crystallised into a firm determination to help the staff.

CHAPTER 3 – PHILOSOPHY AND MODEL OF CARE
INTRODUCTION

85. At an early stage in our work as a Committee we decided that we must formulate and make explicit the broad principles which would provide a framework for our deliberations. We refer to these principles, which we present in the first part of this Chapter, as our philosophy. Subsequently we began to interpret and elaborate upon these principles to provide the substance and texture of the new pattern of care which we feel is required. This we have called our 'Model of Care'. We are convinced that this approach was the correct one. The alternative would have been to begin with a piecemeal examination of particular elements such as training, organisation and manpower which would probably have led us to offer simple but uncoordinated, partial solutions. While strategies for change must be realistic, and changes in professional practice will inevitably be incremental and evolutionary, models and policy objectives can be imaginative and radical. We hope that central government, the various professional organisations and those who provide services to mentally handicapped people and their families will agree that significant structural change of the kind we advocate in Chapters 4, 5 and 6 is needed, and that this change should be the logical outcome of a well thought out philosophy and model of care.

86. *We are equally convinced that these principles and the model must be applied to all mentally handicapped people, including those with very severe intellectual handicap and those who are multiply handicapped.* Too often in the past the concept of "as normal a lifestyle as possible" has tended to stop short of those mentally handicapped people with severe problems. It is still unfortunately assumed that if a mentally handicapped person has additional physical handicaps or severe behaviour disorder he must live in a hospital. But the human rights and needs which we discuss in this Chapter are shared by all mentally handicapped people, however severe their handicap.

87. We have assessed the strengths and weaknesses of current patterns of care, and in particular of professional practice as it relates to residential services for mentally handicapped people against the principles and the model of care contained in this Chapter. We have also used the principles and the model as the basis for our recommendations on training, manpower and the organisation of human resources.

PRINCIPLES

88. During the last decade the care and development of mentally handicapped people and their families have become a key issue in social policy in this country and in many other parts of the world. As beliefs and attitudes have changed towards a minority who, at various times, have been seen as objects of pity or a menace to other people, so societies have marked these changes by making explicit new philosophies. The principles outlined in the 1971 White Paper[2] and in the "Declaration of the Rights of Mentally Handicapped Persons"[23] adopted by the United Nations Organisation in 1971 indicate a growing national and international consensus about the human

rights of mentally handicapped people and the need for action to enable them to enjoy these rights.

89.   As a Committee we have identified three broad sets of principles which in combination underpin our thinking:

(a) *Mentally handicapped people have a right to enjoy normal patterns of life within the community.*

(b) *Mentally handicapped people have a right to be treated as individuals.*

(c) *Mentally handicapped people will require additional help from the communities in which they live and from professional services if they are to develop to their maximum potential as individuals.*

90.   These principles can in turn be interpreted more specifically to give guidance concerning key questions such as: where should mentally handicapped people live, what kind of living environment is required, and how should services be organised?

Living Like Others Within the Community

91. (a) *Mentally handicapped children should be able to live with a family.* The first question to be asked must always be "How can we provide support which will allow the child to continue to live with his own parents and his own brothers and sisters, in his own home, in his own community?" If this proves impossible, we must look first to a long term placement with a substitute family.

(b) *Any mentally handicapped adult who wishes to leave his or her parental home should have the opportunity to do so.*

(c) *Any accommodation provided for adults or children should allow the individual to live as a member of a small group.*

(d) *If they so wish, mentally handicapped people should be able to live with their peers who are not mentally handicapped.* The corollary is that non-handicapped members of the community have a right to grow up and learn to live with their less able fellow citizens.

(e) *Staffed accommodation should wherever possible be provided in suitably adapted houses which are physically integrated with the community.*

(f) *These homes should be as local as possible to help the handicapped person to retain contact with his own family and community.* This means that we need a highly dispersed system of homes. Clustering a number of living units together, whilst it might still allow small group living, would inevitably infringe this principle of *locality* (or localness).

(g) *Mentally handicapped people should be able to live in a mixed sex environment.* For adults this would include the right and opportunity to get married.

(h) *Mentally handicapped people should be able to develop a daily routine like other people.*

35

(i) *There should be a proper separation of home, work and recreation.*

Individuality

92. What about specific extensions of *the right to be treated as an individual?* Here we would list again, as with our explanation of "as normal a life style as possible", but without intending to be exhaustive:–

(a) *The right of an individual to live, learn and work in the least restrictive environment appropriate to that particular person.*

(b) *The right to make or be involved in decisions that affect oneself.*

(c) *Acceptance that individual needs differ not only between different handicapped individuals, but within the same individual over time.* (See for example our pen pictures pages xiii to xvi).

(d) *The right of parents to be involved in decisions about their children.*

Service Principles

93. The two groups of principles (on a normal lifestyle and on individuality) outlined above involve value judgements about the human rights of handicapped people in society. If they are to make full use of these rights and to contribute as members of society the majority of handicapped people will need considerable help – sometimes throughout their lives. It is important that the service system we develop should not be based on historical accident, that it should facilitate rather than hamper the integration of handicapped people into society, and should help the community to accept differences in their peers rather than reinforce prejudices. For these reasons we believe that:

(a) *Mentally handicapped people should use normal services wherever possible.* Special provisions tend to set apart those who receive them and may therefore increase the distance between mentally handicapped people and the rest of society.

(b) *Existing networks of community support should be strengthened by professional services rather than supplanted by them.*

(c) *'Specialised' services or organisations for mentally handicapped people should be provided only to the extent that they demonstrably meet or are likely to meet additional needs that cannot be met by the general services.* Often these specialised services will be required only intermittently or as one component in a more general service. Often the aim will be to provide 'back-up' to a more general service. Wherever possible the special services should be delivered in integrated settings. In the past such services have often been specialised only in name, they have not met defined special needs.

(d) *If we are to meet the many and diverse needs of mentally handicapped people we need maximum co-ordination of services both within and between agencies and at all levels. The concept of a life plan* seems essential if co-ordination and continuity of care is to be achieved.*

---

*A 'life plan' means that for every mentally handicapped individual the delivery of services should be mapped out in advance. At any one time the aims of the present care regime and the options which will be open in the future should be well known to all those involved.

36

(e) *Finally, if we are to establish and maintain high quality services for a group of people who cannot easily articulate and press their just claims, we need someone to intercede on behalf of mentally handicapped people in obtaining services.*

MODEL OF CARE

94.   The model of care which we describe in this section is our picture of what services in the future could and should look like. In this part of our report we attempt to define key elements in a comprehensive high quality service designed first and foremost to meet the needs of mentally handicapped people and their families. We also go beyond the narrow focus of the care of mentally handicapped people in residential accommodation. Although our main recommendations are about the training and organisation of residential care staff we thought it vital to describe the experiences and opportunities needed by mentally handicapped people living in the settings in which we would see them, and the system into which the work of residential care staff would be integrated.

95.   The goals of our model are unashamedly idealistic, and such goals will not be achieved without professional staff, the community, and society as a whole accepting and committing themselves to a very different pattern of services and a very different role in society for the handicapped person. We were aware that it might never be possible to achieve our total model in a world in which financial, social and economic factors change and shift, but we decided that a goal which set out the best possible conditions of care which could be devised should provide the framework for our deliberations. An unattainable ideal can, of course, act as a hindrance to change and action; alternatively it can, at best, give a sense of direction. As our work progressed it became clear that many of the concepts of care which we were discussing had already been introduced in different places and in a variety of forms. From many parts of the world came well attested news of success in the care of mentally handicapped people; we therefore felt that the exercise of drawing up a desirable model of care would be a profitable and exciting one. We are confident that a society which recognises the dignity and worth of its most handicapped members is also likely to develop the most cost-effective pattern of service.

96.   When we compare and contrast our model either implicitly or explicitly with current patterns it is not out of a sense of polemic, but rather to assess where we are at present, and therefore how far we have to progress. We do so also in order to identify strengths in the current system on which we hope the new patterns of care can be built. We are interested, therefore, not only in new goals but also in new strategies. As we have already said, many of the key elements identified in our model of care, and sometimes complete programmes similar to our model, are already in operation in this country and in other parts of the world. To this extent many parts of our model have already been 'tested'. What our model attempts to do is to put these examples together to construct a total picture of what a new service to mentally handicapped people might look like.

Problems in Constructing Our Model

97. Our work was not easy and in visualising possible developments of care, we constantly had to give regard to complex inter-locking factors demanding supple responses from those designing, organising and directly providing care, and also from the community itself. The interrelation between these factors can make it extremely difficult to envisage patterns of care which can narrow the gap between what is needed and what society can, at best, provide.

98. There were a number of other factors which made our work difficult. Neither we nor many of those who gave evidence to us found this 'model building' approach an easy one. Also, much of our work was inevitably based on beliefs and value judgements rather than well established fact. For example as individuals we often found it very difficult not to confuse *our* idea of a small, locally based home with well trained staff and inter-disciplinary 'back-up' with what, from personal experience, we knew about many current community-based homes. Our discussions about the care of those who are most severely handicapped provide a graphic illustration of our difficulties, and indeed of the difficulties facing any group of people attempting to develop new national or local policies. Often these discussions produce conflict. On the one hand there was a group of Committee members who were highly reluctant to approach the task by attempting to categorise or identify "special groups" preferring to view each mentally handicapped person as having needs that might be special in constellation, in intensity, in frequency, or in the complexity of professional response required from both direct residential care staff and from primary and specialist support services. On the other hand, there was another group of members who felt that we were neglecting or ignoring the needs of these "special groups", and that the model of care proposed was one where facilities and professional skills would not be able to accommodate or meet the needs of those who are most severely handicapped. Consequently, they argued, our report would not be credible and, if implemented, would do a serious disservice to many mentally handicapped people and to those caring for them.

99. In the end we had to set ourselves a number of ground-rules. The first was that we would try to avoid a "categorisation of special groups" approach. We preferred to consider each individual as having a unique constellation of general and special needs which were unlikely to be met by trying to match a particular group of residents to a particular kind of building. Instead we agreed that we would look at the professional tasks to be performed, and the kind of *programmes* that would be needed. At the same time, we recognised that there would be individuals who would make very heavy, often lifelong demands on professional services and we found ourselves using the shorthand of "those who are most severely handicapped". Here we must emphasise that this is not a category which corresponds to any one used at present. A second, related ground-rule was that we would view the handicapped person's needs as dynamic rather than static.

100. Thirdly, we wanted to develop an interactive model. That is to say we would construe the handicapped person not as a passive receiver of services but as a person who would make choices about goals for mental handicap and who would interact with others (both professionals and people in the local community). These others would also have needs which would have to be

considered and which could in fact be met by their work or contact with handicapped people.

101. The picture of care which we have constructed tries to follow the course of an individual's life. At each stage it has attempted to cover a range of care from the least intensive to the most intensive. This will not invariably mean that those who are most handicapped will need the most care, nor the converse. The individual, his social circumstances and the degree and type of his disability will all play their part in determining the pattern of care. We have tried to visualise the experiences which mentally handicapped people will need if they are to reach their full potential at each stage in their lives. We have also tried to describe some of the qualities and skills which caring staff will need if they are to provide those experiences.

THE COMPONENTS OF THE MODEL

Prevention

102. To begin with we hope and expect that thoughtful application of the knowledge and technology we already have will, in the longer term, significantly reduce the proportion of children who are born and grow up mildly or severely handicapped. We know, for instance, the importance of good ante-natal care, and the close relationship between the health and behaviour of the mother and the health and development of her child. We are also able to identify those groups of mothers who are 'at risk' with regard to 'pre-term' births. The challenge is to reach and help these and other mothers – such as those who have a higher chance of producing a child with Down's Syndrome.

Support to Families

103. When a child is assessed as mentally handicapped it is imperative that parents get the best possible information and counselling at this sad and fearful time in their lives. Sometimes, the child's handicap will be obvious from birth, but in many children it will be possible to make such an assessment only as the child grows older and it is established that his development is slower than that of his peers. There is evidence that, as professionals, we have mishandled the "telling" (what, when and to whom); that we have been slow to enlist the help of other parents; and that we have often communicated our own prejudice and ill-founded predictions about eventual development rather than offering skilled practical advice on how to meet the child's current developmental needs. In the early years those in the closest contact with parents will be "generalists", such as GPs, health visitors and midwives who have been involved in the ante-natal period, and sometimes also paediatricians and others including nurses and midwives in the maternity and child health services. Attitudes in the professions and among the general public are changing; the general community services are demonstrating their ability and willingness to help mentally handicapped people. This development should be encouraged and the community staff should be offered training to prepare them to work with their new clients.

104. It would be fruitless to list all the general services from which mentally handicapped people could benefit but the Primary Health Care Team (PHCT) of GP, Health Visitor, District Nursing Sister and Midwife will be an important resource for families. The Health Visitor should provide continual support but

the services of other members of the PHCT will be needed at intervals through-out the mentally handicapped person's life. The team has close links with families and is traditionally the first source of help; families with a mentally handicapped member should find in the PHCT a quick and informed response in times of difficulty. We would like to see all members of the PHCT being given additional training in mental handicap.

105. Our model envisages that parents who decide to care for their child at home will quickly find themselves supported by a range of appropriate help, with competent helpers drawn from the whole range of services we have already remarked upon. The important issue is that the support is available, effective and consistent and that it provides a sense of hope. The elements and staff which go to make up this support will depend on what is needed and what is available. The most urgent requirement is for answers to the parents' questions, skilled and compassionate interviewers, health care help and a sense that now and in the years ahead parents will not be alone in facing the care of a handicapped child. Parents themselves speak movingly of their need for practical and emotional support in caring for their children and of their past difficulties in obtaining such help. These problems might be alleviated by the appointment of a specifically named worker. This person, who would be a member of one of the agencies already involved with the family, would be both acceptable to the family and clearly identified by all the other profes-sionals involved. He would be responsible for helping the family to articulate their needs, personally representing them where necessary, and, in co-opera-tion with other professionals, for marshalling the required service.

106. The existing system has often forced parents into making desperate choices: many have cared for their children at home almost entirely unsup-ported, others have found the burden too great and have seen no alternative but to make a complete separation from their child and request for him to be placed in an institution. But already there are encouraging signs that major changes have occurred in the pattern of admission of children to hospitals and other forms of residential care. Those children who do come into long-stay care now do so at a much later stage in life. We think that, in part, this reflects changing professional and public attitudes and beliefs about the best place of care for mentally handicapped children. More important the provision of education as a right to all children has, in our view, made a significant impact on the lives of families with a severely handicapped child, as have some of the new financial allowances.

107. Domiciliary care of the most wide ranging kind may substantially change even further the number of parents who choose or are able to keep their child at home. The active care which we envisage will consist of the most imaginative range of service which can be devised. From the general services will come the best of child care and understanding of the issues facing the parent and child. From the specialist services, the advice and help which gives the parents a chance to take an active part in furthering their child's devel-opment. From the local community networks, the understanding and support which the professionals cannot always provide. Money advice and skilled family counselling may also be needed and there will be occasions when help

40

will be required urgently. The services will include short-term relief of various kinds, providing the parents with a chance to go shopping or to the hairdresser and longer-term relief to allow the family to have a holiday.

108.   We see this type of regular short-term care – which may be for a very short period of time or for a matter of weeks – as a vital element in the support to families. We see other families who do not have a mentally handicapped child as a major and largely untapped resource of short-term carers. The imaginative and flexible schemes in Somerset, Leeds, Northumberland and in other parts of the country encourage us to believe that widespread adoption of this kind of programme is both desirable and feasible. This does not mean that all children could or should be offered this form of short-term care. The small, locally based, staffed house which we describe below (paras 116–117) could also serve a similar purpose, acting as a resource to the local community; so too for certain children could the integrated homes we describe.

109.   The expected benefits of these kind of programmes are considerable. Substantial relief would be available to families who at present receive little or no help. It is anticipated that such care will considerably reduce the stress, on both parents and siblings, which is engendered in caring for the severely handicapped child and will allow them to care more effectively and for longer. Demand for long stay care is likely to be considerably reduced.

110.   An important advantage of short-term care with families, and indeed of locally based homes, is that disruption to the child is minimised and continuity of care maximised. The child will continue to attend his own school and will if necessary be seen by familiar members of the Primary Health Care Team and school health services. More important, particularly with short-term care families, the child will have an opportunity to develop a relationship with the members of his substitute family and this will aid his growth and development. We think that success with short-term 'substitute family' schemes may give professional workers the confidence and expertise required to seek and find long-term substitute families.

Alternative Care for Children

111.   Even with support of the kind described there will be some children for whom alternative homes will have to be sought. On the whole, as we have indicated, these will be older children. At the moment, the main alternative is a mental handicap hospital. We find this quite unacceptable. Our first choice would be long-term care in a substitute home. The substitute parents or professional residential care staff will need much the same order of service as the real parents; it would be sad if substitute care or care in a children's home broke down because it was seen as some final solution which could then be left unattended.

112.   The conditions for the success of such care seem to be:

(a) the availability of a good support system;

(b) opportunity for the training of substitute parents;

(c) a reasonably high financial allowance which takes into account the responsibility and work involved in caring for a severely handicapped child; and

41

(d) a positive commitment and enthusiasm on the part of the social services, local education authority and NHS support staff operating the programme.

113.   Another alternative would be to offer children places in homes where children without handicap live. We realise that if this form of care is to be successful it will require careful attention to the behaviour and needs of the group which the child will join, and to the skills and interest of residential care staff. As with substitute family care it will require good support both from colleagues within the same discipline and from members of an interdisciplinary team. We believe that increasingly children of all degrees of handicap could be accommodated in the normal provision of residential care for children provided by voluntary and statutory agencies.

114.   The needs of a small number of mentally handicapped children will, however, best be met by small, special homes which are locally based. Our preference is for such homes to be in specially adapted private houses. We are beginning to realise the influence of architecture on the nature of the social environment and we need to investigate whether the style of the new purpose-built homes for mentally handicapped people is in fact perpetuating the old "institutional" approach to care. The problems of size and economy of scale will have to be solved. Views on the optimum size of living accommodation for mentally handicapped people have followed a consistent trend in favour of "smallness" in recent years. But whereas a 40 bed ward was regarded as small by comparison with a 70 bed ward 15 years ago, many people now think of "small" as meaning a maximum of 6 children in a house.There is little or no experience of highly staffed homes for 4 to 6 residents and the nearest equivalent, the family group home for disturbed children which was popular a decade ago, is a completely different concept. Our model envisages a home with a small number of residents and an appropriate staffing ratio plus the availability of support from inter-disciplinary teams.

115.   The clustering of a number of units may allow small group living but the very small numbers of children whom we see as needing residential accommodation will inevitably mean that the units could not be truly local. This would make contact with families of children in long stay care more difficult, would hamper the use of the home for short-term care for children in the locality and would restrict some of the outreach work from the home.

116.   The small unit which we envisage is a place where residents and staff live together as a unit, a place where meals are cooked, washing-up is done and tradesmen are seen. In such small homes, whether general or special, the child will experience as normal a life as possible and he will be cared for by staff, both men and women, trained in the care of children living separately from their parents. The home will not be seen as a substitute family, since a key feature will be that the environment is planned to nurture the child while providing him with a group of adults to whom he becomes accustomed and with whom he has consistent (but not constant) close contact and shares a warm life.

117.   In this home the small group of familiar people who care for him will provide opportunities for the child to develop emotionally, by recognising

42

what particularly pleases the child and responding to his personality; physically (by physical contact, cuddling, helping the child to play with special aids, teaching him special exercises); socially (by building up a relationship with the child, helping him to relate to other children and adults, singing to him and giving the child personal attention at mealtimes and bedtimes); and intellectually (by providing general stimulation, creating a stimulating environment and implementing well-designed learning programmes to teach colour, shape, texture and language). The picture we have drawn is one which is needed by all children whether they are cared for in their own homes or elsewhere, but our model requires staff to change their attitudes so as to admit that severely handicapped children can be stimulated and can learn and develop, and it relies on the methods which are now available and are being used to make the special effort necessary to help the mentally and often physically handicapped child to set out on his developmental path.

118. The model we have devised will demand staff who are able to care in these ways and whose duty times are scheduled to offer consistent care. We recognise that staff themselves have a right to duty times which allow them to spend adequate time with their families and to develop their own interests, but we are concerned that each member of staff should be familiar to each resident, and that the work should be so organised that strangers are not suddenly introduced to give intimate care to a child. The staff must be able and encouraged to see each child as someone for whom their whole thrust of care is directed towards the development of all their capacities to the fullest potential. Throughout the working day the well-trained residential care worker should be concerned with the smallest events which are taking place.

119. These residential care staff should have ready access to the specialist advice and help which we have recommended should be available for parents. Once again the contribution of those in the surrounding neighbourhood will be of high importance, and neighbours, shopkeepers and friends will play their part. We want the children to see the milkman and, however small they are, to be taken out shopping. This means that the social unit is one in which the staff are not enclosed but share many aspects of daily living with the children. They must not be bound by routine duties. The leader of the team must have the capacity to devise and run an organisation of this nature and help the care staff to make it work. We have spoken of the help to be sought from general and specialist services; the administration supporting such a home will need to be a flexible one which does not set up structures which take responsibility away from those giving the care.

120. The life of the child in a residential home or in his own home will demand a progression of new experiences. In time children begin to expand their experiences into nurseries or schools; the extent and speed at which this happens will depend on the success and achievement of the earlier patterns of care. Again we visualise a range of possibilities from special care units through special educational provision to normal schools. The debate about special education has been explored by the Warnock Committee and there may well be a growing number of mentally handicapped children and young people to be accommodated in normal schools. One can sketch some of the experiences the developing child will require. He will need experiences which lead him to take an interest in and responsibility for his own appearance and care; to make choices and decisions; to learn social behaviours and skills; to be provided

with changes in regime which give a sense of growing up; to be offered places and times when he can be alone or quiet; to be engaged in a changing relationship with adults which matches his stage of development; to learn a wider sense of the world about him; and the chance to take risks.

121. The question of risk, which at this stage involves such things as climbing and running, and later in life hazards of other kinds, is one of extreme delicacy for those who care. Staff are likely to receive harsh criticisms when accident or injury occurs, yet if we entirely cushion people against these dangers we immediately restrict their lives and their chances of development. This restriction can be cloaked in respectability and defended on the grounds of protecting mentally handicapped people and keeping them safe, but it can also endanger human dignity. Each of us lives in a world which is not always safe, secure and predictable; mentally handicapped people too need to assume a fair and prudent share of risk. As we explain in para 308 each unit should have a well defined policy on risk taking.

122. The details of the picture cannot be developed here. If such a varied experience is to be available, the staff will be of the highest importance. They must have access of the most fluid kind to people and places and be trained to offer the experiences which can augment and extend the care which is offered.

123. Parents who care for their own children will similarly continue to need additional active help from trained people from whom they can learn how to extend the experiences which they can provide for their child. The painful emotions which parents feel need to be relieved by action more often than by counselling. In talking of children in small units away from the parental home we may seem to be taking for granted that there will be complete separation from the parents; clearly this is not intended. We hope for easy and frequent contact between parents and their children who are cared for away from home. This might be through exchanging visits, or by planned and agreed shared care ie with the child living sometimes with his parents and sometimes in a substitute home. We see the necessity for the most active efforts by the residential care staff and those who may be giving other help to the families to make such mixed patterns easily accepted. The importance of involving parents in the life of the residential home cannot be over-stressed. We have too often seen parents drop away from their children because they become strangers to each other. We visualise parents taking part in the daily care of their own and other children and moving easily in and out of the substitute home as an environment in which they can feel entirely at ease.

Adolescents

124. As we continue to look at the stages of life we see emerging a new set of needs for the young person as he or she moves into adulthood, and a new set of demands and challenges for families and for professionals.

125. It is at this time that the mentally handicapped person will need appropriate preparation for the move from school to adult life. This change may be more profound than any he has experienced in his whole childhood and new needs will emerge. Some will be the extension of those begun in late childhood, other needs will be for contacts with peers in their place of residence and outside it; the social networks could play an important part here. Access to youth and community facilities, further education opportunities and leisure

pursuits will be very important. Young people will also need to be freer to engage in activities outside their place of residence and will need experiences which encourage them to occupy their own time. They will need help with their developing sexuality and once again the range of help may encompass learning programmes or behavioural shaping to develop socially acceptable behaviour, or something more akin to counselling in personal and sexual relationships. Meanwhile education, work opportunities and training will be determined by the experiences required by an individual and should be carefully planned by the extensive use of all available resources.

126.   It may be at this time that the individual comes into long-stay residential care for the first time, or that he moves from a children's home to adult accommodation. Again we see a need for staff to be able to prepare the handicapped adolescent for these changes and to be sensitive to the anxiety that he may feel in his new home. We also must prepare parents for the transition of their child into adulthood.

Adults

127.   Our pattern of care leads at different speeds and in different ways forward into adult life. We believe that with the increasing effectiveness of foundation work in the early childhood years, as the mentally handicapped individual moves forward into young adult life the choices open to him or her can be greatly widened. Much of what happens at present is rescue work for those who have not been offered appropriate experiences much earlier in life.

128.   Adult life will present a new set of challenges for the handicapped person, for his family and for society as a whole. Our model requires that the family should not continue to be regarded as the central agent in care and support until parents are old and infirm. We think that the community and the professional services must assume a far greater responsibility than at present. In particular we think that accommodation ranging from highly staffed homes to unstaffed houses and flats should be provided. This would allow the handicapped person to make a choice, jointly with his family, to move on and to establish a life independent of the parental home. This is the normal pattern within our society.

129.   Society is generally less in agreement about the needs of mentally handicapped adults, particularly the most severely handicapped adults, than about those of children. Current policies and practices demonstrate an ambivalence and inconsistency between stated goals and action. It is advocated that mentally handicapped people should lead a life which is as normal as possible, that "adults should not be segregated unnecessarily from other people of a similar age, nor from the general life of the local community", and that the substitute home should be "as homelike as possible". But at the same time policies are developed which assume that large numbers of mentally handicapped adults will continue to live at home until their parents become too aged or infirm, or die. It is argued that large numbers of the most severely handicapped adults who are offered alternative accommodation should be offered places in hospitals, albeit ones serving a district of say 250,000 people. Within hospitals those who are more severely handicapped continue to be grouped together and wards continue to be understaffed with little or no support to the nursing staff. Society continues to talk of handicapped adults as children, to

behave towards them as if they were children and to talk of "meeting individual needs" and "providing specialist treatment" when what is meant is that as a community we wish to segregate mentally handicapped individuals from ourselves.

130. We as a Committee propose that adults – no matter how handicapped – should be treated as adults, and whenever possible provided with the kinds of experiences which their non-handicapped peers enjoy. We realise that this is quite a difficult idea for many people to accept, especially when the handicapped person's developmental level is that of a child. We accept that in some cases it is highly unlikely that a handicapped individual will appreciate the social significance of the actions of those who are interacting with him. We consider it even more important however that the person should, for instance, have clothing appropriate to his age, and to be addressed in a manner appropriate to his age and the social circumstances – in other words that he should be interpreted to others as an adult. We must start to listen to those who are less handicapped talking about themselves. A report of a survey in which mentally handicapped adults living in Wandsworth[24] were encouraged to talk about their experiences, relationships and aspirations provides clear evidence that they are more like us than they are different.

Families

131. Some mentally handicapped people will choose to remain with their families or foster families even when alternative accommodation is offered; we do not envisage that support will be withdrawn from these families. On the contrary they will continue to need help to construct what Michael Bayley[25] in his study of families in Sheffield, has called "Structures for Coping" and "Structures for Living". To these we would add our own "Structure for Development". Families and handicapped people will need the services of counsellors, advocates in obtaining welfare benefits, medical help of general or specialised kinds, advice or help with work, opportunities to be away from home during the day through day centre or other provisions, and encouragement in finding leisure activities. According to the nature of their disability mentally handicapped adults may need encouragement or support to extend their lives outside the home, but profoundly handicapped adults too need to be given the stimulus of active programmes when they are at home. Parents will also need skilled advice concerning teaching goals and methods appropriate to adults. We totally reject the pessimistic view that if handicapped people have not learned important personal and social skills as children they are unlikely to show progress as adults. This belief has no empirical foundation whatsoever. Short-term care will be of vital importance for those families who decide to continue to care for an adult relative. In paras 133–136 we describe a range of local residential accommodation which we expect would be used sensitively for this purpose, as well as for providing a permanent home to other mentally handicapped adults.

Day Care Options

132. There will also need to be a wide range of work and further education opportunities ranging from sheltered employment within open industry to special centres with carefully developed objectives and programmes of the kind described in the National Development Group pamphlet 5.[26] We are

particularly anxious that those who are most severely handicapped should all be offered places and we find it totally unacceptable that someone who has been in full time education should not be offered a place in a community-based programme of this kind. We hope, however, that many more adults will be able to choose where they live and where they spend their day. For those who have grown up in some form of residential care the issues are the same, they will share with their peers who have been living at home decisions about where their adult place of residence should be and how they should live their lives.

Residential Accommodation for Adults

133.　The principles stated at the beginning of this Chapter require that mentally handicapped adults should have the opportunity to leave their parental home. They also suggest that the accommodation we provide should be, in terms of size, design and location, as much like the accommodation we ourselves would wish to live in, but at the same time should meet a continuum of individual need ranging from maximum support and protection to minimal professional involvement in the life of an essentially independent person. In short, handicapped adults must have the opportunity to live in the least restrictive home environment which they as individuals can manage at a particular point in time.

134.　Our present residential provisions in no way conform to criteria such as these. For those who are less handicapped the choice is simply between the parental home or a staffed home in the community, but not necessarily their community. Whilst for the more handicapped the choice is between living with the family or living in a hospital many miles from their home community. This lack of appropriate choice and neglect of individual need is entirely unacceptable to us—we think it is also unacceptable to most handicapped people. Whilst we were encouraged by the imaginative and diverse experimentation which we saw in England, Wales and Scotland, we found no area that could even begin to offer to the 100–200 adults for each 100,000 of the population the range of accommodation which we think is needed. The major challenge in the field of mental handicap is, we believe, to establish a system of residential services for *adults* which goes beyond the family home, hospital ward or local authority home options and provides a high quality service in *each* area. We realise that residential services are the most difficult to organise and that staffed accommodation can be very costly. This is all the more reason why we must develop the most *cost effective* service possible.

135.　Again we believe that ordinary houses, suitably adapted for those with additional physical handicaps, will be needed. Whilst physical integration of accommodation for mentally handicapped people with the buildings in which other people live will in no way guarantee the acceptance of mentally handicapped people, it will, we believe, provide the first step to fuller social integration. A purpose built unit on the outskirts of a housing development or a town is not in our view "in the community".

136.　The principle of small group living, in which most people in our society believe, should be respected. We also want handicapped adults to be offered accommodation that is as close as possible to the social and geographical community in which they have spent their childhood, and perhaps early adult life. This will provide an important sense of continuity through continuing contact with family, friends and familiar professionals. Such requirements – the need for maximum physical integration through the use of ordinary houses, the need for small living groups, and the need for localness are not met by large purpose-built homes or by concentrations of handicapped people in one place. Whilst the highly dispersed and differentiated network of residential accommodation we advocate will bring with it new problems, its advantages will be considerable.

Independent Living

137. What kind of options do we visualise? First we expect that in the future many more people who are mentally handicapped will live in flats and houses which they themselves have rented from local councils, housing associations or private landlords, or in houses which they or their families have purchased. This they may do as single people, as married couples, or in small groups. We know from our own experience how successful this kind of truly independent living can be. In many parts of the country the opportunity to move into an unstaffed group home has allowed the handicapped person to develop the confidence and the ability to initiate a move beyond supported accommodation into truly independent living.

Group Homes

138. For others, placement in an unstaffed but supported group home will represent the maximum kind of independence that they will be able to manage. Here we want to emphasise that we have no set ideas about what constitutes a group home – it may involve two people or it may involve five. Similarly we would wish to emphasise that this is not an option which we see as appropriate only for the most able. We have been very impressed by the imagination of those staff who have been willing to give handicapped people, some of whom may have been in hospital for very many years, a chance to move into this kind of home. Often in a mixed ability group one member is able to complement another in terms of household management or personality. For a person who has lived in staffed accommodation for many years, where he or she has had to make few decisions, and interpersonal difficulties with friends have often been 'solved' by staff members, living in a group home can initially be a source of great anxiety. At the same time it can provide an opportunity for the development of skills that have remained latent for decades. Some homes may involve a lot of visiting from highly skilled staff whilst others will require infrequent visiting. The amount of support that a particular group needs may vary over time and flexibility must be built into our programme. The first solution to the problem of an individual who is not doing too well should not be to look for an alternative placement in a staffed home. That should be the last. Making homes of this kind work will demand a lot from support staff. Institutional approaches of the kind described by King, Raynes and Tizard[27] are not confined to institutions. They can emerge in professional practice in the community. Even though an agency may hold the rent book or own the home, we see the residents having the major say in who comes in and leaves their *home*. Where there is incompatibility amongst members of the group,

the provision of a number of such homes may allow groups to split up and reform spontaneously.

139. One interesting development of the group home idea, which we believe could allow more people to live in this way, involves the employment of a staff member to live in close proximity—perhaps in the house next door. This would allow more regular on-going contact than is likely to be possible from visiting support staff. It follows that we do not see group homes as either a cheap or an easy option but one that has tremendous advantages for many mentally handicapped people who are currently living quite inappropriately with their parents or in staffed NHS or local authority accommodation which has a degree of supervision which they do not need.

Accommodation Shared with Non-Handicapped People

140. We also see the sharing of accommodation with non-handicapped people as an important element in our continuum of residential care. This could take a number of forms. We are, for instance, aware of programmes in this country and abroad where non-handicapped people contract to share a house or flat with one or two mentally handicapped people. As with the substitute family schemes we have advocated for children, it seems entirely acceptable that a financial allowance should be made available in return for friendly supervision and support. One of the major advantages of this kind of shared accommodation is that the handicapped person lives in close proximity and can learn by example from his non-handicapped peers. Another option would involve living in a home or boarding house or boarding out with a family. We must emphasise that we are not talking about boarding houses in cities or coastal towns where large numbers of mentally handicapped people are congregated for financial gain. Such arrangements do not represent a significant improvement over large minimally staffed wards or homes. This is not what we mean by community care. Finally we envisage that some mentally handicapped adults as they grow older will be able to enter sheltered housing schemes.

Staffed Accommodation

141. It is clear that many mentally handicapped adults will need considerably more help than could sensibly be offered by the kinds of accommodation we have described above. But are the choices currently available to these people acceptable? We have already indicated that they are not. In particular, we cannot support policies on the provision of residential care which attempt to distinguish, on the basis of degree of handicap and/or degree of personal and social adjustment, those mentally handicapped people who need care in community based homes, and those who need hospital care. Our OPCS survey indicates that local authority homes tend to accommodate only the more able adults. We do not wish to deny that many mentally handicapped people will need very intensive and highly skilled staff support, nor that some mentally handicapped adults will be unresponsive or difficult and that interactions with them may often be unpleasant and may bring little direct reward to the staff caring for them, but our model requires that the residential accommodation which we offer to the more severely and indeed profoundly handicapped people should conform just as closely to the principles we have described as

would the accommodation for those who are less severely handicapped. In other words the accommodation should be small, should serve a local community and, wherever possible, should use suitably adapted ordinary houses. The homes we envisage should also be capable of acting as a resource to the families in the locality.

142.   These staffed homes would allow for people with varying degrees of intellectual handicap. Each home would be for men and women and would be staffed by men and women. We cannot hope to help mentally handicapped people to acquire normal behaviour patterns unless we can provide examples of normal behaviour and relationships. Too often in the past we have compounded the problems of handicapped people and of those caring for them by grouping together those with similar handicaps and denying mentally handicapped people the possibility of learning from each other *and* helping each other.

143.   As with the children's homes we would envisage meals being cooked in the house and residents having personal space, with individual bedrooms (except in the case of those who expressly wanted to share their sleeping accommodation with someone else). The climate of experience for adults, depending on their personal, social and physical development, would be one in which personal competence and personal identity were continually strengthened; in particular, in making decisions, as much freedom as possible would be normal. The practicalities or difficulties involved in making it possible for mentally handicapped adults to decide when to go out and when to return, who they should be friends with, how they should spend their money and what they should eat would be seen by residential care staff as exciting problems to be solved, rather than barriers to progress.

Specialised Staffed Homes

144.   We found no valid reason for a distinction between "treatment" and "residential care" since in our thinking an active developmental programming is required by mentally handicapped people with all degrees of handicap and all kinds of problems. Nor, in practice, did we find persuasive evidence that the accommodation currently provided, which is separate from the community, is in most cases meeting the identifiable and justifiable needs of handicapped people or of the community. There were, however, members of the Committee who argued that even the well staffed local homes described in our model would not be able to meet the needs of a small minority of mentally handicapped adults and children, those who we have described elsewhere as 'the most severely handicapped'. This might include a small minority of those who are profoundly handicapped and who also have associated physical and/or sensory handicaps and those with very severe behaviour disorders whether mildly or severely intellectually handicapped.

145.   The arguments, as we have already indicated earlier in this Chapter, are complex ones. The rights and needs of individual profoundly handicapped people to live in the most normal environment possible have to be finely balanced with the needs and rights of their handicapped peers to enjoy a life that is not continually disrupted. Similar considerations also apply to the community and to residential care staff.

146.   Those who favoured separate more "specialised" short and long term accommodation for 'the most severely handicapped' argued that:

(a) The staff in the local homes would be more likely to accept the more severely handicapped and difficult residents and to try to help them if they knew that there was a "back-up" residential service available.

(b) Unless specialised homes were planned from the outset with appropriate staffing levels and with staff who had the right kinds of skills and experience such homes would emerge spontaneously as "dumps" for the most difficult residents.

(c) Without such specialised accommodation staff would be unlikely to develop the special skills required and new techniques for modifying socially unacceptable behaviour and stimulating unresponsive people would be unlikely to develop. The experience needed to meet special needs would be gained only through continuing contact with particular problems.

(d) It would be possible, through transfer of a resident to such a unit, to modify his behaviour successfully so that he could then return and live successfully in his original home.

Against this it was argued that:

(e) The availability of such "back-up" units would of itself encourage staff in the ordinary units to give up too easily when faced with a difficult resident and to "pass the buck".

(f) Moving a client from one home to another could actually create additional problems of adjustment for the handicapped person.

(g) Grouping the most severely handicapped people together, even given an appropriate staffing level, was unworkable and would probably lead to low morale in these units.

(h) Difficult behaviour which might emerge in one of the local homes might not do so in the specialised unit. Similarly, new behaviour learned in the specialised unit would not necessarily be carried back to the person's "home".

147.   In the end we agreed that our model would encompass the possibility of some small specialised residential accommodation. This would have to be provided on a regional or sub-regional basis – for instance a home for profoundly handicapped blind–deaf people or a home for seriously anti-social mentally handicapped people. Wherever possible these homes should share as many of the characteristics of normal living which we envisage in our staffed local homes as possible. Again we saw little merit and many disadvantages in clustering a number of specialised homes on a single site. Where separation from the community and a degree of security are needed these should, if possible, be provided through staff; the siting and design of accommodation should augment this rather than compensate for lack of staff or lack of skills.

148.   We believe that those planning services at a local level should be required to justify any request for specialised accommodation and the nature of the care programmes to be offered should be clearly defined. When an

individual was considered for placement in such a home the expected benefits should be clearly stated, the programme to be provided clearly described, and the progress of the individual regularly reviewed. In all cases where an individual was identified as having a special problem the first response should be to attempt to deal with that problem *in situ*. Those people transferred into specialised homes should be taken back into their own "home" as soon as possible. Since there is so little documented empirical evidence on the need for and effectiveness of such specialised homes we urge that appropriate research programmes be undertaken. We believe as a matter of principle that the onus is on those who believe in such specialised programmes to demonstrate their value.

Elderly Mentally Handicapped People

149.   In the later years of life the problem of age will be added to the problems of mental handicap. In the future, more people with a mental handicap are likely to survive to a greater age. It is hard to tell how many severely mentally handicapped people will live on to old age, but some caring Units will be required for these people. Questions of retirement, admission to suitable accommodation and the right to live at home are problems which society must face for all elderly people and the solutions should benefit mentally handicapped old people too. We hope that more and more elderly people who are mentally handicapped will have recourse to normal provisions and services and that many of these people will be so well established in their way of life that they can move smoothly into their old age.

The Residential Care Staff

150.   The model presents issues which must be further developed and poses questions to which answers must be found. The first among these is this: What sort of worker in residential care could help to make the model a reality and what will be expected of such a worker? Those who gave evidence to us found it hard to express what the tasks of the residential care worker consisted of, except in very broad terms. The analysis of professional work to be done, undertaken by the Health Care Evaluation Research Team in Wessex[28] was, however, very useful to us in our deliberations. Our model envisages a growing number of mentally handicapped adults and children resident in accommodation not especially designed for them. There must clearly, therefore, be some attitudes, behaviours and skills common to all residential care staff working with all possible groups of clients. For both specialised and general skills we will be describing a cluster of attributes which should be available among staff rather than trying to designate levels of accomplishment or responsibility. There is no doubt among us that residential care staff should receive training which helps them to feel confident in their professional world and provides them with the sense of belonging to a respected group in society.

151.   The first general attribute required is one which is hard to define because it has so often been hidden by professional roles, large organisational systems, inadequate expectations of individual staff or rigid specifications of the role to be filled. It is the quality of naturalness or individuality and freedom from restricted ideas of one's self in a post, role, hierarchy or profession. (The study by King, Raynes and Tizard[27] develops this idea.) Its absence has led to

criticisms of training and of professionalism and the demand for what could (impertinently) be called a "back to nature" approach. We understand some of the despair which has given rise to these criticisms but think this despair is unfortunate. We believe that the naturalness and spontaneity of the residential care worker can be left intact by training and that the additional knowledge, skills, sensibilities and intelligent thought which good training brings can help to create a caring person who would himself be nurtured by the model of residential care which we postulate. Our model demands just such people; who are able to be themselves and who can allow their residents to be themselves; who are willing to accept their role as a very open one to be developed as the circumstances demand; whose warmth of care has few conditions attached to it; and who are able to care for people who may be dependent without falling into the trap of kindly control. The image may appear superhuman on the page but we have met people in hospitals and homes who get it right most of the time, and many more in whom this spontaneity struggles to get out from behind the formal role imposed on them.

152. The staff will also need a belief in the capacity of all handicapped people to move forward, and a sense of their own contribution to this process. We recognise that at our present state of knowledge a few mentally handicapped individuals are unable to make significant or perceptible developments. Although their numbers are small such people still need respect from those who care for them. The residential care staff will need help from others to sustain them in their continued attempts to reach these profoundly handicapped individuals; the ability to keep trying will be the important thing. The whole thrust of the model is towards this end; if the structures which make it possible are lacking, residential care staff will not be able to sustain their buoyancy but will fall back into the routines by which we defend ourselves against anxiety and hopelessness. We must not forget that it is just as easy for the staff of an institution to cease to be individuals and to become subordinate to the collective life of the whole; like the residents whom they care for they need to see themselves as individuals, and be treated as such. Only recently has attention been drawn to the professional depression of nurses in the "back wards" of mental handicap hospitals[29, 30]. The staff themselves do not always recognise this depression but it can be seen in the staff of homes and hospitals. One manifestation of "professional depression" is the lack of care of staff for one another and their failure to respond to each other's achievements, often through lack of encouragement, support and advice. If we can get the structures right, and if the staff can be given knowledge, skills, clear tasks and responsibilities and a sense of hope they should develop the wide ranging approach which our model demands. They would then enjoy responding to individual challenges and helping to make decisions in the changing interests of those to whom they offer care.

153. With all mentally handicapped people, but particularly with those who are the most dependent, and whose development is likely to be minimal, we would expect staff to understand the importance of "presenting" these people to others in the most normal way possible. Staff should, for instance, realise the importance of attractive and appropriate dress, hair styles etc, and of correct forms of address which help others to realise that "John Smith" is a person.

154.　Among the other attributes of residential care staff should be the capacity to make the environment agreeable and relaxed and yet at the same time appropriate to the age of the residents. This is really not a difficult goal to aspire to; sadly we often fail to reach it in our present institutions. But we have seen a hospital ward which, by imaginative co-operation between ward sister and residents, had been turned into a comfortable sitting room with footstools, low lamps and ornaments; it was rare. We also saw the rich texture in ornaments and personal treasures built up in their bedrooms by residents in an unstaffed home, and the merry chaos in a small local authority home as children were put to bed in a house of splendid untidiness. The personal care of residents will range from the services which any homemaker would provide (seeing that there are clean socks) to much more demanding personal care which individuals will need because of the nature of their handicap or the stage of their development. Some of this work will be dirty or distasteful; we would be unhappy if a group of residential care staff emerged who saw their work entirely in terms of educational or social development programmes and who were "above" the bodily necessities. Happily this does not seem to be happening and training must take great care not to change it.

155.　Engagement is a word which is often used to describe a concept of care which goes beyond merely keeping the residents warm, safe, clean and well fed. We are not merely in favour of engagement, we regard it as an essential component of our model, but we feel that there is a danger that the word is becoming a hollow term. Our model does not envisage engagement at all costs. Part of the skill of the residential care staff will be in recognising peaceful and contented inactivity and in discovering from the residents (if necessary by asking them) what activity they would prefer to be engaged in. The imposition of knitting or other well meant devices on a group of otherwise idle residents may be done with good intentions but it is no substitute for a good knowledge of the resident's likes and dislikes.

156.　Above all each residential care worker must be able to learn to plan and take part in whatever developmental programmes are designed for individual residents. This will be the medium through which the resident's maximum potential is developed. The understanding and observation of residential care staff will play a significant part in the design of the experiences for people of all ages. We have seen the imagination and patience which a young, untrained worker in a Scottish hospital brought to making contact with very young babies. She used music, rhythm, touch and colour to reach the children and delighted in their small responses; she was greatly sustained by the pride which her nursing colleagues took in her work. The residential care staff will develop a store of understanding, skill and behaviour which it seems wasteful to contain within the residence itself. We hope that these staff will become part of the network of provisions so that they can transmit their knowledge and achievements to workers in other non-specialist units and to the families who are caring for mentally handicapped people at home.

157.　To complete our model we need to focus on three important concepts. The first concerns an individual life plan for each handicapped person; the second, the need for a specialist inter-disciplinary team which can provide a back-up service to the residential care staff; the third concerns parental involvement.

An Individual Plan

158.   We have stated as a basic principle that mentally handicapped people have a right to be treated as individuals. We have also recognised that meeting individual needs is not to do with finding a category or label for the individuals and linking it with a matching facility within existing services. Rather we believe that it is to do with clear identification of needs within each individual and the careful development of a programme in which general and special services are appropriately balanced and co-ordinated. Each mentally handicapped person's life should be assessed at regular intervals and key questions should be asked:

What needs to be done in this situation, at this time?

Where, how and by whom should it be done?

How is the work of several people to be co-ordinated?

How is progress to be evaluated?

Inter-Disciplinary Teams

159.   It follows from our beliefs about the needs of mentally handicapped people, the way in which they vary from one person to another, and the way in which the needs of an individual will change over time, that no single profession could possibly begin to provide a total service. Instead, our model envisages a network of services within which certain professionals may, through close personal contact, come together, sometimes as a generic team, for instance as outlined in the Court Report[31], or at other times in a more highly specialised form of team, for instance a Community Mental Handicap Team.

160.   If professional staff, parents and substitute parents are to live and work with mentally handicapped adults and children they need the support of inter-disciplinary professional teams. The members of these teams would come from many fields and would probably include experienced residential care staff, nurses, occupational, speech and physio-therapists, social workers, psychologists and psychiatrists, but should not be limited to these people and should be constituted according to local needs. The team members would work across administrative boundaries without status-seeking or tension. They would bring their advice, knowledge and skills to the assistance of residential and day care staff. They might be called in to observe a particular behaviour problem which the residential care staff could not cope with or to advise on a suitable programme. The aim of the teams' interventions would be to ensure that residential care staff were not left with problems which they did not understand. Members of the team might also take an active part in therapeutic endeavours. We envisage a two-way traffic whereby the residential care staff themselves would be called on as experts in certain circumstances.

161.   This idea is not new and has often been promulgated, but it has not been systematically exploited. One speech therapist or psychologist on his own can give a very limited direct service, but by planning and advising on remedial programmes to be carried out by residential care staff and reserving his own direct skills for the most difficult cases he can reach many more clients. But, on the other hand, external professionals will not be able to work effectively without skilled observation and teaching ability on the part of the residential care staff. This kind of inter-disciplinary co-operation has rarely been achieved

even amongst the most highly trained professionals. The new reponsibilities and roles which we want to encourage in residential care staff will make new demands not only on them but also on the members of back-up teams who may feel professionally threatened. We hope that a primary concern for mentally handicapped people and their well-being will over-ride these concerns and that there will be mutually advantageous change and development amongst complementary professions.

A Partnership with Parents

162.   When decisions are being made about the future of a mentally handicapped person it is important that, wherever possible, both he and his family should be fully involved and in agreement with the final decision. It is not sufficient to assume that professional staff, however well trained, automatically know what is best. Mentally handicapped people should be offered expert advice on future care and treatment by professionals with specialist knowledge of the facts and the prognosis of the case; they would then be able to accept or reject this advice in the normal way. Staff will need to accept that they are advisers as much as residential care staff and that parents have a right to be involved in decision making. In the past it has often been difficult for families and staff to make contact; families have felt (with or without justification) that they were outsiders. Some have lost contact with their children, not for selfish reasons but because they could find no place for themselves within the scheme of care. It has been suggested that families who have seemed to drop away have re-established their links when their mentally handicapped relative has been placed in a smaller, more informal setting, nearer to home. Two moving comments, made by mothers at the recent opening of a local home in which parental involvement is actively encouraged, illustrate this point: "No one will ever take away the gift of kissing my daughter, Victoria, goodnight again" and "It is almost like having my daughter back home again. I feel as though I nearly lost her".[32]

163.   Staff and families need to forge new links based on a new concept of the role of residential care and of residential care staff. We believe that staff can derive a great deal of satisfaction and personal reward from working with families, who should be able to turn to them as a first source of help in their difficulties. Staff have much to offer in the way of interviewing and counselling skills and a knowledge of where to go for advice and help on mental handicap and general welfare matters. The importance of involving families in the life of the unit cannot be over-stressed. We envisage parents taking part in the daily care of their own and other children, and moving easily in and out of the home.

CONCLUSION

164.   It is from the principles and the model of care described in this Chapter that our recommendations about training, manpower and organisation have been developed. Taken together, as they must be, we believe they form the basis of a new deal for all mentally handicapped people and their families and for those who provide the care. *But to achieve our vision will*

require major new initiatives and commitment at both local and national level over and above that already shown over the last few years.

165. We have *not* considered it appropriate to make recommendations about how our model should be introduced; we consider that to be a job for others. We are however convinced that the complex pattern of residential services within the community which we propose could not be implemented without the continued involvement of both social services departments and NHS authorities. The majority of severely mentally handicapped people who are not at home are, at present, living in hospitals, many of which are large and remote and lack almost all of the characteristics which are fundamental to our model. We do not suppose that these establishments can disappear overnight. Indeed, we recognise that if they did the plight of mentally handicapped people would be considerably worse than it is at present. *With all their defects, these buildings are places in which many dedicated people are providing love, care, training and support to clients who desperately need those things. It is the staff in these hospitals and the staff in the local authority homes who have begun to show the way in which our model of care could begin to be implemented today.* We discuss in the following chapters the changes which we see as necessary and the ways in which they can start to be made now.

CHAPTER 4 – MANPOWER

INTRODUCTION

166. *It was clear to us from the start that the type of care which we envisaged for mentally handicapped people would require many more care staff than are employed in this field at present.* Our model is one of active care and the OPCS survey shows that a poor staff ratio leads to staff having to spend their time giving "basic care" (feeding, washing, dressing and toiletting the residents) rather than encouraging the residents to do these tasks for themselves. (OPCS table 35.) It is not enough, however, simply to say that more staff are required, we also had to consider how many and what type of staff were required, how they should be deployed and how they might be recruited.

Number of Staff Required

167. To estimate the number of mental handicap residential care staff who would be required we had first to estimate the number of mentally handicapped people likely to need residential care in the years ahead.

Estimating the Client Population

168. We were asked to work within the framework of the policies of the 1971 White Paper, but we share some of the doubts which have been expressed about the validity of the planning guidelines in "Better Services for the Mentally Handicapped". Since the White Paper was published estimates of the general population have been revised and the proportion of mentally handicapped children to adults has proved lower than expected. In addition, as we explain in para 169 there is no satisfactory method of determining appropriate staff/resident ratios. In the absence of reliable information on both sides of the equation (ie demand for residential accommodation and demand for staff) it is impossible to make exact calculations of future manpower requirements. We therefore decided that it would be unproductive to spend time devising a sophisticated staffing formula; instead we have made the best use we can of such information as is already available.

Calculating Staff Ratios

169. Some guidance on the way staff ratios might be calculated would have been very helpful to us as a basis for discussion of our own staffing philosophy. But it quickly became apparent to us that such guidance as was available related mainly to the care of clients other than mentally handicapped people. Unfortunately the report "Residential Care—Staffing and Training"[33] produced by a Working Party of the Social Services Liaison Group was published too late to be of use to us. Nonetheless we looked at the "Aberdeen formula" for calculating nursing staff establishments in general hospitals; the Castle Priory Report "Residential Task in Child Care"[34]; the DHSS minimum standards for staffing in mental handicap hospitals; and the formula used to calculate staffing requirements in the Sheffield Development Project hospital units for mentally handicapped people. We also considered the possibility of finding an existing residential unit run on similar lines to those advocated in our model of care. We decided against this for 3 reasons: (1) it would be difficult to find such a unit; (2) the number and level of staff required in any one unit would vary according to local circumstances and needs; and (3) our model of care is not a blueprint to be followed slavishly in all circumstances

but a set of guidelines to be interpreted flexibly, so that we would need a variety of examples to illustrate different interpretations. We *RECOMMEND* **however that once our model of care has been put into effect its manpower implications should be subject to continuing monitoring and evaluation.**

170. Since there is at present no satisfactory formula for calculating staff ratios, or even estimating roughly what they should be, we decided to look at the problem afresh. We used our own experience and subjective judgement to decide on a collective view of a reasonable staff/resident ratio at which our model of care could be carried out satisfactorily. To do this we tested 2 different sets of assumptions and compared the results. The first of these we have called the dependency group method because it is based on staff/resident ratios which vary according to degree of dependency; in devising this method we have drawn heavily on the Castle Priory Report. The second method makes no distinction between degrees of dependency and is similar to that used by the DHSS in planning staff ratios for the Sheffield Development Project. *We do not recommend either method and indeed there are aspects of both methods which go against our model of care; we have simply used these two methods to test the results, in terms of manpower requirements, of working from two quite different hypotheses on staffing ratios.*

Dependency Group Method
Classification of Groups
171. For the dependency group method we considered various ways of assessing the groups and finally decided on the classification of residential groups used by the OPCS in their survey for us. This divided adult units into four categories: high ability; average ability; low ability; and non ambulant with very low ability, according to the characteristics of the residents. Children's units constituted a separate category and were mainly low ability, or non ambulant with very low ability. We are aware that these are not discrete groups and that there is some overlap between them, but for the dependency group method it was necessary to determine some sort of categorisation, however arbitrary, in order to estimate future manpower needs.

172. For this method of calculation we had to make a number of assumptions about the residential care of mentally handicapped people. These assumptions do not always represent our own views on, for example, how a mentally handicapped person should spend his waking day, but merely set out the factors which would affect the staffing calculation.

Waking Day of Residents
173. We based our calculations on a longer day than is usual in mental handicap residential care. This is in keeping with our philosophy of allowing mentally handicapped people to lead as normal a life as possible since it would provide time for a greater potential choice of activities, although it would also require increased staff. We have assumed that some residents, especially those of high and average ability, might be up as early as 06.30 and some might go to bed as late as 23.30, (21.00 in the case of children). Those at work might be away from the unit at any time between 07.30 – 18.00 on weekdays, while others might be absent between 09.30 and 15.30 or 16.00 (except during school holidays, for children).

59

Waking Night Staff

174. We identified a number of reasons why waking night staff might be required: to help residents in time of sickness and distress; observation; help and action in emergency; on-going caring needs. For the least dependent adults (ie a proportion of those in the high ability group) we assumed that waking night staff would not be required, although there might be a need for staff "on call". For the rest of the adults in the high ability group and the whole of the average ability group we assumed there would be a need for some waking night staff, who might be shared between different units on one site. For the low and very low ability group adults we assumed a need for 1 waking night staff member to 15 residents, with an additional member of staff on call. For all children we assumed a ratio of 1:12 with an additional member of staff on call.

Number of Residents Cared for by One Care Worker

175. Under this dependency group system one residential care worker would be able to look after a larger number of low dependency residents or a smaller number of high dependency residents (but see para 181 for other views on this concept). We have assumed the following ratios of staff actually on duty to residents present in the daytime for the purposes of the model:

	Staff : Residents
High ability adults	1:6
Average ability adults	1:5
Low ability adults	1:3
Very low ability adults	1:2
Very low ability children	1:2
All other children	1:3

In practice, if a unit were to be staffed according to this method, various factors in addition to dependency would have to be taken into account in the calculation of staff ratios. These factors, which would need to be assessed locally, include size of unit, organisation of living group(s) within the unit, and degree of staff involvement with the residents.

Number of Residents "At Home" During the Day

176. Ideally all residents would be out of the unit during the day – except at weekends and during holidays – attending education or occupation and training centres, or in employment. In practice there will almost always be somebody who has to stay in the unit because of illness or for other reasons. We have therefore included an allowance of 25% in our daytime manpower estimates (roughly equivalent to a 10% increase in total care staff manpower requirements) to allow for daytime care.

Staff Holidays, Sickness and Training

177. We have included an allowance of 25% to cover staff holidays and sickness and in-service and post-basic training. This allowance is based on experience of nurse staffing, increased slightly to allow for the extra time away from residents which would result from our recommendations on in-service-training for Basic Care Staff. (See Chapter 6 for the explanation of our proposed new staff grades.)

Hours of Work

178.   We have used the basic 40-hour week.

Contribution to Service by Trainees

179.   Under our training proposals (see Chapter 5) Trainees taking the qualifying training would spend approximately 50% of their time on theoretical work and supervised practice and 50% at work in residential and other units. During the 50% work element of the training a Trainee would not be fully productive and we have therefore estimated that each Trainee adds the equivalent of 25% of a full-time Basic Care Worker to the workforce.

Other Factors

180.   There are other factors which affect staffing requirements about which we could not make any useful assumptions. These factors include:

involvement by senior staff in training of junior staff;

staff deployment at peak hours;

work with families outside the units;

a margin for contingencies;

the direct care contribution of Unit Heads;

implications of long and short term care.

The Sheffield Method

181.   The first model we have described is based on the grouping of mentally handicapped people according to degree of dependency – defined in physical and behaviourial terms. The alternative model takes no account of dependency and could therefore be used to calculate staff complements in units for residents with any degree or type of dependency. The degree of dependency of the residents is ignored on the grounds that the more able, less dependent, resident requires well thought-out educational and social training programmes which are just as demanding on staff time as is the perhaps more physical care required by the less able, more heavily dependent person. We have called this staffing model the Sheffield method since it is based on the criteria used to determine staffing levels in the residential units of the DHSS Sheffield Development Project.

182.   The Sheffield method assumes that all mentally handicapped people in residential care need a family-type therapeutic environment, as similar as possible to that of a non-handicapped person living at home. Thus adults and children are assumed to have somewhat different needs, with children requiring close individual care from a semi-permanent staff and adults needing more independence and being allowed more scope for self-help. The ability of staff to respond to these two types of need would depend on such factors as the size of the living group and the staff/resident ratio. In all cases, however, *at least* two care staff would be required for any one group of residents since one member of staff would be engaged in one-to-one relationships and the other would be relating to the rest of the group. There is very little researched evidence on the optimum size of living groups and attendant staff ratios. The Sheffield Development Project Feasibility Study[35] recommended groups of 8 residents for children and 12 for adults. Using the Sheffield figures we allow, in this model, for ratios of 1:1 for children's units and 1:1.5 for adult units;

(we have made allowance in the staff total for changes in the working week). This would ensure the availability of 2 care staff per unit during the daytime, plus night-time cover.

Reservations About Our Calculation Methods

183. We have already explained our reservations about the White Paper estimates of need for residential places, and about the two methods of calculating staff numbers which we have used. Both methods rely on subjective judgements and contain inconsistencies which we could not exclude. Additionally there were many variables of which we were unable to take account, including:

> number of independent living units on one site;
> number of living groups within these units;
> number and mix of residents;
> staffing pattern according to size and lay-out of unit;
> shift arrangements;
> mix of grades and of sex of staff;
> number of staff in training;
> impact of changing patterns of care.

All these variables are important in estimating local manpower requirements, but we were more concerned with arriving at a national picture of the number of residential care staff required. We used the dependency group and Sheffield methods simply in order to establish the order of magnitude likely to be involved and to test how far this was affected by the use of different methods of calculation. We do not suggest either method as appropriate for national or local planning purposes nor do we wish to suggest the adoption of the staffing patterns on which our illustrations are based.

Results of Our Calculations

184. In the event both the models we tested produced remarkably similar results – both demonstrating a requirement for about 60,000 direct residential care staff (for England, Scotland and Wales). This congruence between the results of the two methods of calculation gave us some confidence that we were working on the right lines, but no certainty that the figure produced was anything more than a very broad estimate of the number of staff which our model of care might require. The figure of 60,000 staff relates to the White Paper planning guidelines of about 74,000 residential places for mentally handicapped adults and children (approximately 62,000 places for adults and 12,000 places for children). There are currently (1976 figures) about 28,500 direct residential care staff to care for about 60,000 mentally handicapped children and adults. **We thus** *RECOMMEND* **an approximate doubling in the numbers of the mental handicap residential care staff** (that is those in direct contact with residents) although there would in any event have been some natural growth in nursing and residential care staff numbers. In the future direct residential care staff would consist of qualified and in-service trained staff; the current figures include trained nurses, nursing assistants and learners and qualified and unqualified staff in local authority homes.

185. The reservations with which we have had to hedge our calculations do not render the results completely useless. The calculation confirmed what

we had always expected: that our philosophy and model of care would be expensive in terms of manpower. *There can however be no halfway measures; our model requires not only that staff should be trained in the best techniques of residential care, but also that they should have the time to practise them.* This is important for self-help programmes where it is often quicker for staff to do things themselves than to teach and assist the residents to do them. Any attempt to provide a cheap solution by employing fewer care staff than we recommend would result in a reduction in that standard of care which we believe is not only necessary but the right of every mentally handicapped child and adult. Maureen Oswin, in her study "Children Living in Long-Stay Hospitals"[29] has produced striking examples of the professional depression and poor standards of care which inevitably result when trained staff are prevented from practising their skills. **We therefore strongly *RECOMMEND* that health and social services authorities press ahead towards the staffing target of 60,000 direct residential care staff which we have proposed, as fast as their finances will allow.** Improvements in staff ratios have been continuing since 1965 and our recommendations are simply for an acceleration of that improvement. Our recommendations are of course only broad national figures and individual authorities will need to estimate their own staffing needs within our guidelines. Because of the scale of the increases which we are proposing, the lack of agreement on optimum staffing ratios need not deter field authorities from embarking on large scale recruitment programmes; authorities would be unlikely to reach the position where residential services for mentally handicapped people are "overstaffed" within the forseeable future.

DEPLOYMENT OF STAFF

Problems

186.   Staffing any form of residential establishment is made difficult because of the peaks and troughs in activity which occur throughout the day; small units are particularly subject to this difficulty. We have assumed the peak demands to be early in the morning; late afternoon and evening; and weekends. A number of methods have been devised to overcome this problem, most of which involve variations on the shift system including:

the "long day" (ie 12 hours);
overlapping early and late shifts;
6 short shifts making up a full week;
the use of part-time staff.

It is clear from our OPCS survey (para 2.3) that part-time working up to and including Staff Nurse level is an important element in the manpower equation of current mental handicap hospitals.

187.   Problems with staff deployment and solutions to these problems are often dependent on local conditions; a unit situated in a rural area will have different problems from those of a unit in the middle of a large town. We are therefore unable to propose any universal solution to the problem of uneven manpower needs throughout the day and individual authorities and their staff must devise their own systems which will best suit their local needs.

Peak Hours

188. We do however wish to comment on the consequences of some particular solutions to staffing problems. Long day working has been severely criticised in previous reports and while there is no need to restate the objections we too are opposed to this system. We are also not in favour of split shifts and although adequate overlap should be allowed to provide for a proper hand-over between staff long overlap between shifts should be avoided. This should apply particularly on weekdays at times when some or all of the residents are away. Long overlaps may be acceptable, however, in order to provide for in-service training, or to prepare for recreational or other activities with the residents. *The peak hours of early mornings and evenings require maximum staff cover.* At these times there will be many tasks suitable for Basic Care Staff to perform (such as bed-making, serving breakfasts) and the assistance of regular part-time staff will be most welcome. But the daily routines of getting up and going to bed have important implications for the individual programmes of the residents and provide important opportunities for self-help programmes; experienced staff at all levels should take an active part in care at these times of the day.

Weekends

189. For mentally handicapped people as for everyone else the weekend should provide an opportunity for recreation, relaxation and the development of both new and old interests and activities; it should not be, as it so often is, a period of boredom and stagnation. To this end *sufficient staff should be deployed at weekends to ensure that both staff and residents can participate in enjoyable pursuits both inside and outside the residential setting.*

Daytime

190. *We believe that work experiences and living experiences should be separate for mentally handicapped people just as they are separate for most other people.* Spending 24 hours a day, 7 days a week in the same building or group of buildings, so that work and leisure are found in the same place, contributes to the isolation and institutionalisation of mentally handicapped people, no matter how cheerful the surroundings. Ideally residents should leave the home unit each weekday and spend the day at work, at school or at a training, social or other activity centre. This does not mean that the residential care staff will be left idle. We have already explained (para 176) that some residents may have to spend the day "at home". In some instances staff from the day centre may visit the unit, in which case the residential care staff will need to be on hand to assist; in other cases residential care staff may accompany residents to the day centre. But on those occasions when all the residents are out, or there are more staff available than are needed by the residents then in the unit, there are still a number of important tasks for residential care staff to carry out. These include staff training, administration, family support, and group work with families, all of which might be arranged according to local needs. Apart from going out into the community to give family support, residential care staff might provide short-term day care within the unit for mentally handicapped people living at home. This day care would be for specific purposes, such as intensive social training or to provide relief for

64

parents, and would be strictly limited so that the residents' privacy was not abused by the use of their bedrooms or personal possessions.

Continuity

191.   It is in the interests of staff morale as well as of continuity of care that staff should have a regular, permanent work base. *It is detrimental to the well-being of the residents and to the efficiency of the unit if staff are frequently taken away from their own unit or living group to fill-in elsewhere because of staff shortages.* It is therefore essential that the Head of the Unit should make contingency arrangements to cover for staff sickness or other emergencies. *One solution is to maintain a register of people who would be willing to do a spell of full-time or part-time work in an emergency.* These arrangements are intended to apply to Basic Care staff and qualified staff; Trainees would of course need to move within and between living units to obtain experience.

Liaison with External Professionals and Relatives

192.   *Residential care staff should work closely with other professionals – including the primary health care team, psychiatrists, psychologists, the remedial professions and social workers – and with the domestic staff of the unit.* External professionals and residential care staff should work together to prevent isolation of the unit and to ensure full multi-disciplinary care. To this end external professionals should make regular visits on a planned basis. These visits should be arranged to suit the needs of the residents and residential care staff should regard working with outside specialists as an important aspect of their work. External professionals should never visit without the knowledge of or in the absence of the residential care staff and each visit should include discussion with relevant members of the residential care staff about the outcome and implications of the visit for the individual resident concerned.

193.   Parents and other relatives will be among the most important visitors to the unit. They should always be made welcome and involved in discussions about their relative's needs and progress. We were impressed at one unit we visited to find that families were free to visit at any time; there were no formal "visiting hours" and all those involved – most of all the residents – told us they found the freedom of contact rewarding. Time spent with families must be allowed for in the deployment of staff within the unit.

Staff Leisure

194.   Increasingly staff prefer to work regular and fixed hours and they should not be expected as a matter of course to sacrifice their own interests by working long, inconvenient or additional hours, particularly at short notice. *Residential work with mentally handicapped people is physically and emotionally tiring and staff should be able to get right away from the work-place and live their own private lives when the work is done.* This is not merely a matter of good personnel relations: staff who are overtired and completely immersed in their work lose their objectivity and cannot give the best care to the residents. Management should be sensitive to staff needs and should find imaginative solutions to particular problems of staff deployment. The organisation of the unit, though putting the needs of the residents first, should not make unacceptable demands on staff.

DAY CARE

195.   We believe that mentally handicapped people should wherever possible find their leisure activities in general recreation facilities rather than in the residential unit or ATC. **We similarly** *RECOMMEND* **that responsibility for the day-time activities of adult residents during the week should be with staff trained to teach mentally handicapped people.** This is already the case for all mentally handicapped children, who must be taught by trained teachers, and for those adults who attend Adult Training Centres where they are instructed by specially trained staff. We have said that ideally all residents should leave the unit during the day; where this is not possible specialist day care staff should visit the unit just as special school teachers visit hospitals to teach mentally handicapped children who are unable to attend a school.

196.   At present, day-time activities during the week for adults in hospital are often organised by the ward nurses. Under our model these activities would be the responsibility of specially trained staff and there would thus be a need to increase the number of students taking the day care training (the one year Diploma in the Training and Further Education of Mentally Handicapped Adults which is being replaced by the Certificate in Social Service). The OPCS survey shows (Table 31) that 5% of nursing staff work in a variety of occupational, recreational or training centres. This would mean that approximately 1100 nurses are employed in this work at present and therefore at least 1100 day care staff would need to be recruited to take on the job.

197.   Apart from the need to recruit trained day care staff, residential care staff too would be needed to look after those people who could not, for various reasons, go out to a day centre and who would therefore be visited by day care instructors. According to recent DHSS statistics as many as 30% of hospital residents do not attend day care activities, for reasons which include "severe mental and/or physical disability" and lack of facilities. We believe that our model of care will reduce this percentage considerably as residents benefit from increased attention from a larger number of staff, but we have nonetheless included an allowance in our manpower calculations to cover those residents who stay "at home" during the day (see para 176).

RECRUITMENT

198.   Having estimated how many residential care staff are required and considered how they should be deployed we had to consider how they could be recruited. Figures 7–9 show the recent trends in mental handicap staffing in the health and social services. Figure 7 also includes numbers of residents in mental handicap homes and hospitals to illustrate the trends in staff/resident ratios. It is not, however, possible to make reliable comparisons between mental handicap nursing statistics from the NHS and mental handicap residential care staff statistics from local authorities. The nursing figures include administrative and tutorial nursing staff some of whom may have little or no direct contact with the patients. In the local authorities on the other hand, ATC staff, teaching staff (employed by the local education authority), study supervisors and senior staff not based in a home are all excluded from the residential care staff statistics.

FIGURE 7: – STAFF (WHOLE-TIME EQUIVALENTS) AND RESIDENTS IN HOSPITALS AND HOMES FOR MENTALLY HANDICAPPED PEOPLE (ENGLAND, SCOTLAND AND WALES)

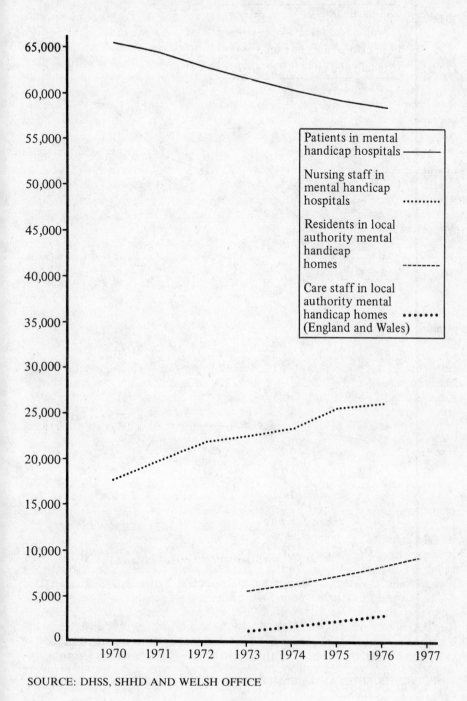

SOURCE: DHSS, SHHD AND WELSH OFFICE

FIGURE 8: – NURSING STAFF (WHOLE-TIME EQUIVALENTS) ON MENTAL HANDICAP HOSPITALS (ENGLAND SCOTLAND AND WALES)

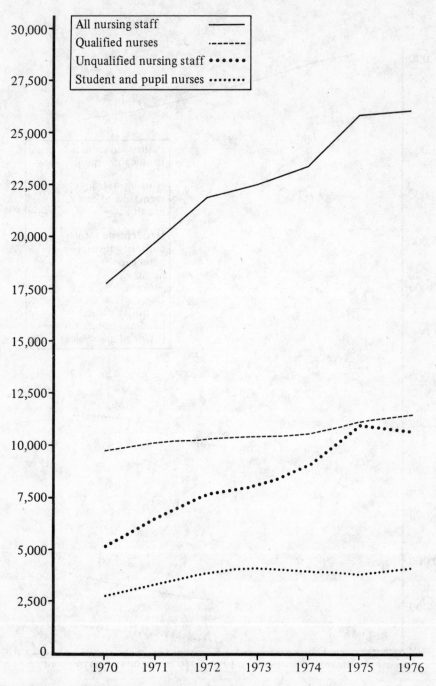

SOURCE: DHSS, SHHD AND WELSH OFFICE

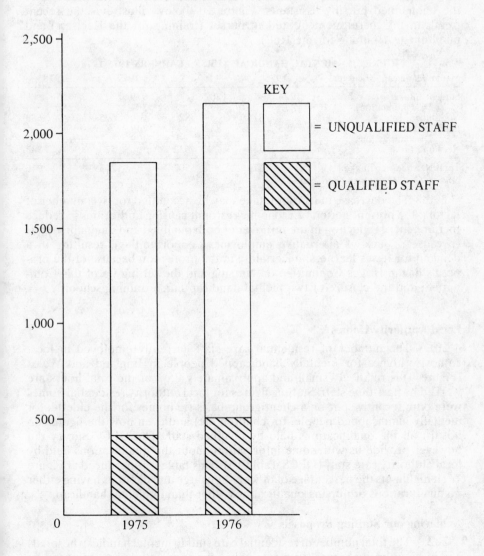

Note: In considering these figures of full-time staff it must be remembered that local authorities make great use of part-time staff; for example in 1976 there were 1033 part-time care assistants in England and Wales, equivalent to 578 full-time staff.

SOURCE: DHSS AND WELSH OFFICE

69

Mental Handicap Hospitals

199.   Figure 7 shows that increases in the number of mental handicap nursing staff have coincided with a small but continuing reduction in the number of patients to produce an improving staff/patient ratio. Figure 8 however shows that the increase in staff is almost entirely accounted for by the unqualified nursing assistants. Figure 10, below, illustrates the recent trends in the recruitment of student nurses (training for the Register) and pupil nurses (training for the Roll).

FIGURE 10 – MENTAL HANDICAP NURSE LEARNERS 1975-1978

Mental Handicap – Learners	1975		1976		1977		1978	
Student Intake	1224		1202		979		815	
” Discontinuations	413		332		304		257	
Net Student Intake		811		870		675		558
Pupil Intake	695		852		749		545	
” Discontinuations	230		220		179		157	
Net Pupil Intake		465		632		570		388
Total Net Learner Intake	1276		1502		1245		946	

Source: GNC for England and Wales.

200.   The decrease in learner intake may be accounted for by a number of factors: the present period of economic restraint causing authorities to reduce recruitment; a reduction in the turnover of both qualified and unqualified staff (because of lack of alternative employment opportunities), resulting in a demand for fewer learners; uncertainty in the profession because of the proposals of the Briggs Committee on Nursing and the setting up of this Committee; and the closure of two mental handicap nurse training schools.

Local Authority Homes

201.   The number of residential care staff currently employed in local authority homes for mentally handicapped people in England and Wales (Figure 9) is relatively small and approximately 25% of the total hours are worked by part-time staff. Staffing figures for local authority residential homes were only recently split on a client group basis (ie homes for the elderly, for mentally handicapped people, for children etc) and even now the figures do not list all the qualifications held by qualified staff. The OPCS Survey did however provide us with some information about the qualifications held by local authority care staff (OPCS Table 16). This table is reproduced at Figure 11; it highlights the percentage of officers-in-charge and deputies having either no qualifications or nursing qualifications other than in mental handicap.

Achieving our Staffing Proposals

202.   The total number of residential care staff in mental handicap hospitals and local authority homes for mentally handicapped people has increased by almost 50% since 1970 but within that total the number of qualified staff has increased at a much slower rate. *To achieve the manpower targets which we have recommended will require a massive build up of learners to provide the 50% qualified work force which we are advocating (See Chapter 6) and a less dramatic increase in the number of in-service trained staff.* In the following paragraphs we consider how new groups of people might be attracted to mental handicap care.

70

AVAILABILITY OF RECRUITS

203.   Examination of population projections produced by the Government Actuary in "Population Projections 1975–2015",[36] and labour force projections 1971–1991 in "Employment Gazette"[37] confirm that the age structure of the work force is changing. Figures 12–14 show that the numbers in the 16–19 age group will increase steadily to peak around 1981–3 and then decline until 1996–2001 after which they will pick up again. In the 30–54 age group numbers will increase steadily to reach a plateau around 1996–2006 after which they will decline steadily.

FIGURE 11 – NURSING AND SOCIAL WORK QUALIFICATIONS OF HOME STAFF BY GRADE

	All Home Staff	Officers in Charge	Deputies	Other Care Staff
	%	%	%	%
Summary of qualifications:				
Has obtained qualification(s) in both social work and nursing	2	10	5	0
Has obtained qualification(s) only in social work ..	10	25	15	6
Has obtained qualification(s) only in nursing ..	15	31	24	10
Has no formal qualifications in nursing or social work	73	35	56	84
	100	100	100	100
Type of social work qualification obtained:				
CQSW—professional social work qualification (Certificate of Qualification in Social Work)	1	2	2	1
CRSW—(Certificate in Residential Social Work)	5	17	5	2
CRCCYP or SCRCCYP—(Certificate or Senior Certificate in the Residential Care of Children and Young People)	5	9	12	3
DipTMHA—(Diploma in the Training and Further Education of Mentally Handicapped Adults) ..	1	4	2	0
NNEB—(Nursery Nurse Education Board certificate)	2	4	3	1
Type of nursing qualification obtained:				
RNMS*—(Registered Nurse for the Mentally Subnormal)	5	15	10	1
SEN(MS)*—(State Enrolled Nurse for the Mentally Subnormal)	3	10	3	1
SRN*—(State Registered Nurse)	3	9	7	1
RMN—(Registered Mental Nurse)	5	17	5	2
SEN(M) or SEN*—(State Enrolled Mental Nurse or State Enrolled Nurse)	5	3	5	6
Base for percentages all home staff (reweighted)	324	115	59	216

Source: OPCS Survey, Table 16.
*Or equivalent Scottish qualification.

FIGURE 12 – POPULATION AGE STRUCTURE—GB, IN THOUSANDS

Age Group						1978	1982	1996	2006
17–19 yrs	..	..	..	..	..	2,532	2,754	1,884	2,571
30–49 yrs	..	..	..	..	..	13,305	13,696	16,016	16,035

Source: Government Actuary—"Population Projections—1975–2015"[36].

204. The implications of these figures for our manpower model are clear: in the 1980s and 1990s the usual source of recruits to trainee grades—the 16–19 year olds—will be on the decline, but there will be increasing numbers of men and women (including a large number of married women) in their 30s, 40s and 50s—the age group from which nursing and care assistants have traditionally been recruited—available for work. We see no reason why this should create problems for recruitment of Trainees, indeed *there are consid-erable advantages in a Trainee grade which encompasses both school leavers and more experienced people.* The training structure we propose is flexible enough to adapt itself to recruitment from a variety of sources.

Resource Implications

205. It is clear that the speed at which staff numbers can be increased will depend to a great extent on the finance which is available; decisions on recruitment are therefore matters for political judgement. Since there are currently more unqualified than qualified staff it would be possible to achieve a rapid increase in staff numbers comparatively cheaply by bringing Basic Care Staff numbers up to their target (30,000 staff) and then starting on Trainee recruitment. We reject this proposition because we wish to see the 50/50 balance between qualified and Basic Care Staff, on which our model depends, introduced at the earliest possible opportunity. **We therefore** *RECOMMEND* **that, if there is to be any special drive on recruitment, expenditure should be focused on Trainees,** since there is a significant shortage of trained staff at present. In Chapter 7 we consider the financial implications of our recommendations and propose various strategies by which our manpower targets could be reached. *We wish to make it clear, however, that our model of care depends crucially on the availability of many more staff than are employed in the care of mentally handicapped people at present.* If sufficient resources are not made available care staff numbers will remain at a level where often only the most basic custodial care is possible.

FIGURE 13 – GB PROJECTED TOTAL POPULATION, AS AT MID-YEAR, BY AGE 1975–2013—BASE MID 1975

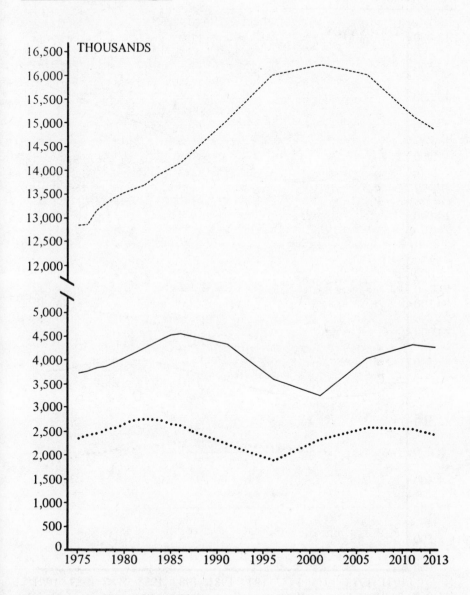

No. of 17-19yr olds ········
No. of 20-24yr olds ————
No. of 30-49yr olds ---------

THOUSANDS

SOURCE: GOVERNMENT ACTUARY

73

FIGURE 14 – GB LABOUR FORCE PROJECTIONS (EXCLUDING STUDENTS) AS AT JUNE, BY AGE, 1971–1991

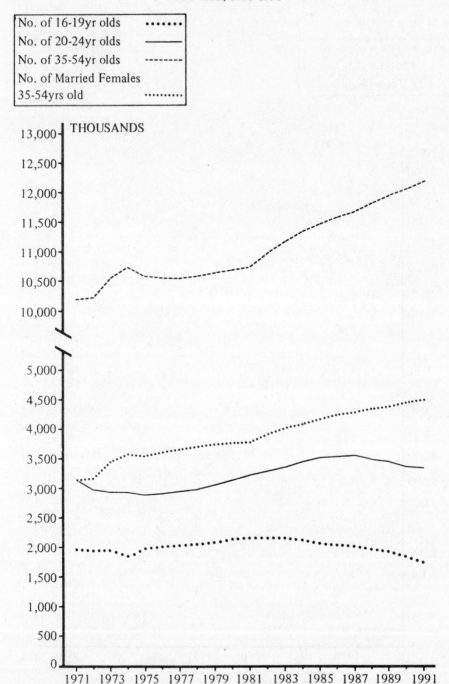

No. of 16-19yr olds	••••••
No. of 20-24yr olds	——
No. of 35-54yr olds	-------
No. of Married Females 35-54yrs old	••••••••

SOURCE: DEPARTMENT OF EMPLOYMENT GAZETTE. APRIL 1978.

Male and Female Staff

206. Although in recent years there has been a much freer integration of male and female staff, particularly in hospitals, the OPCS study shows that existing staff are predominantly female (70% female, 30% male). Figure 15 below shows how the proportion of male and female staff changes at higher levels.

FIGURE 15 – SEX OF NURSING AND HOME STAFF

Sex	Senior Nursing Staff	Ward Sisters	Nursing Assistants	All Nursing Staff	Officers in Charge	Care Assistants	All Home Staff
Male	70%	50%	16%	30%	45%	7%	18%
Female	30%	50%	84%	70%	54%	93%	82%

Source: OPCS Table 3.

It is inherent in our concept of a family pattern of care that residents should be able to relate to both male and female staff. We believe that our proposed new caring profession will offer the opportunity of an equally worthwhile career to both sexes and we hope that broadly equal numbers of each will be recruited. When it comes to part-time staff, whom we see as continuing to make a considerable contribution to the work force, we have however to accept that women are likely to outnumber men mainly because part-time work is particularly attractive to women.

Recruiting

207. We believe that our model of care is not only essential for the care of mentally handicapped people but also has many features which should make it attractive to potential recruits. Chapter 11 of the OPCS report provided us with information about the attitudes of current staff towards their careers. Staff with less than 6 years' experience (ie 59% of all nurses and 69% of all local authority home staff) were asked their reasons for choosing to work with mentally handicapped people. It is true that in their replies the staff may be reflecting their current attitudes to the job as much as their initial reasons for taking up mental handicap care, but the results are none the less interesting. Table 85 of the survey shows that only 23% of recently recruited nurses gave as their main reason for taking up mental handicap nursing "wanting to do (or continue doing) a nursing job". By far the largest group—48%—mainly wanted "a job that involved caring for people". The considerable increase in staff numbers which we propose would permit staff to play an active thera-peutic role in the care of mentally handicapped people. Our recommendation that direct residential care staff at all levels should have more independence and be given more responsibility would raise their status and allow them to operate on equal terms with other professionals, (indeed, we see the Unit Head as taking the leading role in inter-disciplinary decisions affecting resi-dential care). Our concept of informal small group living with encouragement of individual initiative is, we believe, more attractive than a large hierarchical organisation run by uniformed staff. Future recruits to mental handicap resi-dential care would know that under our proposals they would receive a training which would prepare them appropriately for their active role. This training would also enable them to gain experience either in residential care with other client groups or in other work with mentally handicapped people with a minimum of additional training.

208.   *We think that there is scope for interesting more people of all ages in residential work with mentally handicapped people and to this end more and better publicity is required at both national and local levels.* This publicity should provide information about mental handicap itself and about the residential care of mentally handicapped children and adults. The Central Office of Information films on nursing are a good example of this type of publicity. Measures should be taken to recruit staff locally as well as nationally and use should be made of such facilities as the local press, visits to local schools, open days, and the parents' association as means of interesting people in mental handicap residential care. *There should also be a drive to inform careers advisers in schools about the opportunities for work in this field at Basic Care Worker level as well as in the qualified grades.* Careers advisers should know about the availability of qualifying training for suitably qualified 18 year olds, and the possibility of qualified school leavers working as Basic Care Staff until they can take the qualifying training at 18. Those who leave school without suitable qualifications should know about the formal in-service training which we propose for Basic Care Staff and the possibility of experienced but unqualified Basic Care Staff moving on to qualifying training. *Different recruitment strategies will be needed to attract older staff and efforts should be made to encourage recruitment among men and women looking for a change of career in middle life.*

Retaining and Attracting Back Staff

209.   Recruiting staff is of course only half the battle: once recruited they must be retained. People leave their jobs for a variety of reasons, some of which are avoidable, others not. The ordinary sequence of life (marriage, pregnancy, retirement), moving to another district or spouse changing jobs can all result in unavoidable wastage. The desire for a change, a personality clash or straightforward disillusionment with a job can also result in staff losses, but in these cases wastage can be reduced by good staff management and welfare services. For our manpower calculations we had to assume an element of wastage and the figure we used was based on past experience, mainly in nursing; but the features which would make our model of care attractive to new recruits should also help to persuade existing staff not to leave.

210.   In addition to the inherent attractions of our model of care we also wish to see conditions of service improved in other ways. *There should be good counselling and welfare services for staff, with advice and help available on both career and personal problems. Creches for young children would help to encourage mothers to return to work, as would flexibility in duty hours. There should be enlightened industrial relations and personnel policies and each unit should have an operational policy based on participation of staff at all levels.* All staff should be encouraged to join the appropriate unions and professional associations. Efforts should be made to keep in touch with women who have left to bring up their children and who might return to residential care work later. These people might be encouraged to join the list of "emergency helpers" (see para 191). Staff who have left might be encouraged to keep in touch through newsletters and invitations to join seminars etc arranged for serving staff.

76

CONCLUSION

211.   We believe that with determined efforts on recruitment publicity many new groups of people will see mental handicap residential care as a new and exciting career prospect offering a highly relevant training, good staffing levels and a flexible and democratic management structure.

CHAPTER 5-STAFF TRAINING

INTRODUCTION

212. In this Chapter we explore the training demands of the model of care set out in Chapter 3. We consider the organisation and content of the training required by those who will give residential care to mentally handicapped people. For the majority of mental handicap care staff – the nurses – we are recommending far-reaching changes in training; for the local authority mental handicap residential care staff we are proposing significant but less radical changes. Inevitably such changes will involve a period of upheaval; we believe that the best way to minimise the hiatus is for an early decision to be taken on our proposals. We have therefore suggested some practical solutions to the problems thrown up by our model in the hope of facilitating a speedy implementation of our report.

213. In Chapter 6 we describe the various levels of skill required in a residential unit. We describe the work to be done by the Basic Care Worker (who would roughly equate to the present Nursing or Care Assistant) and the Qualified Care Worker. In this Chapter we describe the qualifying training required for the Trainees who will become Qualified Care Staff and the in-service training required for the Basic Care Staff. We also make recommendations about post-basic training for Basic and Qualified Care Staff.

THE TRAINING DEMANDS OF OUR MODEL OF CARE

214. We decided to tackle the problem of what training should be provided for the Trainee who will become a Qualified mental handicap residential Care Worker by looking at the needs not of the staff, but of the residents. We went back to our model of care (Chapter 3) and considered the knowledge, skills and attitudes which it demands of staff. For example, having decided that mentally handicapped people should be free to take risks as part of normal life it is clearly important that residential care staff should know what kinds of decisions and judgements people with different mental handicaps could be expected to cope with at different stages of development. This implies that staff should know about the many aspects of mental handicap and about how the handicapped person develops. We decided that we would build up a picture of the sort of people we wish to see caring for mentally handicapped people. We would expect the body responsible for the training to translate our picture into appropriate curricula for mental handicap residential care staff.

THE MENTAL HANDICAP RESIDENTIAL CARE WORKER

215. The individual who is to work with mentally handicapped adults and children should be motivated to help others to achieve their full potential and should be willing to take on a very demanding job. He will need an appropriate education, training and experience to develop his sense of responsibility and maturity. His job will involve communicating both with the residents and with other staff, and, more importantly, articulating the needs of his clients where this is necessary. The residential care worker should be patient and willing to work with individuals who may never give much or indeed any sign of social

response in return. In his work he will need to understand the sort of responses he can expect from his clients and also the extent of development which he can work towards with different types of handicap. For this he will need a general understanding of mental handicap in all its forms. He will also have to understand and to cope with the health and behavioural problems which mental handicap frequently entails. His training should therefore cover the basic health problems associated with mental handicap and the common behaviour difficulties, and how to treat them. On the other hand the residential care worker should consider his clients as individuals, balancing "What can this person achieve?" against "What are this person's limitations?". His training should therefore focus on human development of all kinds rather than on the isolating abnormalities of handicap. There is always the possibility of an adverse response to mental handicap by the public and the residential care worker will have to help the local residents in his area to understand the problem. He should know, or know where to find out about, all the services which are available to mentally handicapped adults and children: from the financial benefits provided by central government, through the facilities and advice provided by local health and social services authorities to the help which local and national voluntary bodies can give. Thus his training should provide up-to-date information on services and how to make the best use of them.

216.   The residential care worker's most important job will be to teach his clients to help themselves. He should be able to help mentally handicapped children and adults to learn how best to look after their own physical needs – feeding, washing, toiletting, dressing – but often he will have to see to these tasks himself. Though the aim should always be to work towards greater independence for the client, some mentally handicapped people will, at least initially and perhaps indefinitely, need skilled and intimate physical care simply in order to survive, let alone to develop. The residential care worker will need to be both knowledgeable and versatile in identifying for individuals at very different stages what is their next step towards independence and how to help them make it. Part of the residential care worker's job involves making a home for his clients and he should make use of this activity for social training purposes – eg by taking the residents out shopping, helping them to wash their clothes and involving them in keeping the house clean and tidy. We recognise that teaching a mentally handicapped person even the simplest task is time-consuming and requires patience; initially at least it is always quicker to do the job oneself. Staff who are overworked cannot be expected to help and encourage residents in the way we have described. But our manpower model provides sufficient numbers for residential care staff to take pride in teaching self-help rather than in doing tasks for the residents. The residential care worker's training should therefore equip him to teach mentally handicapped people these practical tasks. In his work he will need an understanding of group, family and individual dynamics so that he can create an atmosphere in which mentally handicapped people can learn the skills, behaviour patterns and social responses which most people acquire throughout childhood and adolescence. Working within a team he should be able, and above all have the time, to play a full part in devising and implementing a treatment programme for each of his clients so that each resident is involved in a continuing scheme of active care. As well as teaching his own clients the residential care worker

will have to assist in training junior staff and may also have to advise and assist parents and other relatives looking after a mentally handicapped person at home. He should therefore not only understand the concepts of care but also be able to explain them clearly and simply to others.

A COMMON TRAINING FOR HOSPITAL AND LOCAL AUTHORITY STAFF

217. In drawing up our picture of the "ideal" mental handicap residential care worker we started with the needs of mentally handicapped people. We had to decide whether mentally handicapped people in hospitals had different needs from mentally handicapped residents in local authority homes. Eventually all those needing residential care should be catered for by locally based accommodation, but for some time to come there will be people whose real need is for residential care in a small, locally-based Unit but who, because of the scarcity of this type of accommodation are cared for in hospital. Some people assume that mentally handicapped people can be divided between those who need residential care – to be provided in local authority homes – and those who need nursing care – to be provided in mental handicap hospitals. Others believe that the hospital "patient" could not be offered the "normal" lifestyle which is being developed in the homes. But it is generally agreed that there are a number of hospital "patients" who could be transferred to homes if the places were available. Indeed our survey shows (OPCS Table 24) that two-thirds of adult wards in mental handicap hospitals contain residents of average or high ability and that half of these residents had an ability level similar, so far as basic skills are concerned to the residents in the locally based homes and hostels.

218. Thus it is quite possible that one-third of adult wards contain "patients" who would be able to cope with life in a home. Clearly these people have the same needs and rights as their home-resident peers. *But we believe that all mentally handicapped people, whatever their degree of handicap and wherever they live, share the human needs and rights which we discussed in Chapter 3.* The characteristics of the residential care worker we have described are those needed by staff working with all mentally handicapped people in residential settings, though each client will require an individual approach based on his personal needs at the time. We have stated our belief that residential accommodation for mentally handicapped people should be provided – whether by health or social services authorities – in small units, or homes. These units would be staffed by residential care workers. But we recognise that the mental handicap hospitals will be with us for many years to come and in Chapter 6 we discuss the need for large institutions to be reorganised as federations of semi-autonomous, small living groups. Throughout our report the term "small unit" is intended to include these reorganised hospital wards. Having formed the view that all mentally handicapped people in residential care need the same range of knowledge, skills and attitudes in the staff who care for them it seemed to us illogical to perpetuate separate systems for training staff to meet that need. **We therefore** *RECOMMEND* **that mental handicap residential care staff in the health and social services should receive a common training.**

80

TYPE OF QUALIFYING COURSES

219.   In paragraphs 215 and 216 we described our ideal care worker in terms of training needs. We envisage these needs as being met initially through the training courses for the Qualified Care Staff though we also stress the importance of continuing education throughout the working life to develop fresh skills and up-date existing ones (see paragraph 254). Basic Care Staff would not undertake a qualifying training but would receive a formal in-service training as described in paragraphs 255-256. We explained in paragraph 214 that we did not wish to draw up detailed syllabuses for training programmes. Our objectives in considering training for the Qualified Care Staff were:

a.   to define the outcomes we expected from the training, and

b.   to specify the particular features which we considered essential to the training.

220.   The main outcome we expected was that the training should produce the knowledge, skills and attitudes required for the "ideal" worker. Additionally the training should facilitate the inclusion of mental handicap care within a general residential care profession, made up of specialists in the different fields of residential care. (This is discussed further in Chapter 6 paragraphs 275-278). We wish to see mental handicap residential care staff as part of this wider grouping because our model of care shows that many of the features of good residential care are not specific to mental handicap. Our model of care suggests a programme for training residential care staff with the accent on caring for mentally handicapped people rather than a programme for training mental handicap care staff with the accent on the residential setting.

The Specialist Component

221.   What we regard as the essential features of our training programme derive from this concept of a general residential care profession. We believe that much of the knowledge and many of the skills required for the residential care of mentally handicapped people are common to all forms of residential care but also that there is a significant combination of knowledge and skills which is uniquely required by those who will work with mentally handicapped people. The care of mentally handicapped people requires an inter-disciplinary approach and residential care staff need support and expert assistance from a variety of professions. But just as a parent over the years learns how to be nurse, psychologist, teacher and social worker all in one, so to a greater extent the mental handicap residential care worker must achieve a basic minimum level of understanding and competence in a variety of skills. Each of these skills, taken individually, might be the basis of specialisation of a profession, but it is the combination of particular aspects of these skills which is unique to the mental handicap residential care worker. We *RECOMMEND* **that mental handicap residential care workers should undertake a training which will provide for both the generic residential care and the unique mental handicap care components of their work. These two elements should be covered in both theoretical and practical work.** We would hope that the training body will hold extensive consultations with interested parties to define the training requirements. For the generic component students should gain both practical and theoretical experience with client groups other than mentally handicapped people.

81

Care of Adults and Children

222.   **As part of the qualifying training we** *RECOMMEND* **separate modules for those who will work with adults and those who will work with children and adolescents. These modules should include both practical and theoretical elements.** The modules could be included in either the specialist (mental handicap) or the generic (residential care) components of the training.

THEORY AND PRACTICE IN TRAINING

223.   It was suggested to us in evidence that one of the disadvantages of the current nurse training was that the learner nurses were regarded first and foremost as employees. The question of whether Trainees should be students or employees is linked with such problems as who should select staff and students, whether training should be full-time, part-time, "sandwich" (ie block-release) or day-release, and who should pay for training. We considered that in tackling these problems we should start by looking at the type of training we wanted and work forward from there. *Our model of care involves the acquisition of knowledge and skills which would require a balance of college-based theory and unit-based practice.* This does not, however, mean that all theoretical teaching would be college-based and all practical work unit-based. Although it would be for the training body to work out the operation of the basic training we consider that the two elements of theory and practice should occupy approximately equal time and importance during the training. For students to obtain experience with more than one client group and with both hospital and local authority units practice placements would have to be in a variety of locations. **We therefore** *RECOMMEND* **that qualifying training should be full-time, with equal periods of theory and practice.**

RECRUITMENT AND STATUS OF TRAINEES

224.   We considered two basic methods of recruitment for those who would become Qualified Care Staff, firstly recruitment direct to training and secondly recruitment by the employing authority with secondment to training. Under the first system applicants would be able to go straight into training without any previous experience, while under the second, employers would normally expect at least one year's service before secondment. With secondment the employer is able to select staff on the basis of aptitude for the job, whereas a college would be primarily concerned with ability to profit from training. It has been argued that direct recruitment to training leads to the eventual selection of staff who are intellectually able but not necessarily good at the job. Nevertheless, even with training via secondment employers have to consider an applicant's academic ability since colleges are not bound to accept staff put forward for training. Conversely, under the system of direct recruitment to training, authorities are not bound to employ all those who have completed their training, although with a shortage of trained candidates authorities would clearly be under pressure to do so. Advocates of the secondment system argue that the pre-training experience which it requires ensures that training is not wasted on people who, once they start work, find they do not like the job. On the other hand potential recruits to the Qualified Care Worker grade might be unwilling to spend an unspecified time working

as Basic Care Staff before they could be seconded. *We believe that the best solution is a merger of the two systems in the form of a Trainee grade.* The applicant would be appointed as a Trainee and would be assured of secondment to the qualifying training within a specified period – perhaps 1 or 2 years, though it could be as soon as he entered the grade, particularly where a health authority was the employer. The Trainee would still have to fulfil the requirements of the college providing the training; if he could not satisfy their entry requirements he would be removed from the Trainee grade. Basic Care Staff would of course be eligible to seek qualifying training at any time; indeed we regard it as an important function of managers to seek out and encourage training potential among the Basic Care Staff. We would expect colleges to look favourably on such applicants whose motivation was proven and whose experience should enrich their own and fellow students' learning. Although we favour the Trainee grade we recognise that it may not always be appropriate and that some applicants may prefer to enter training direct. **We therefore RECOMMEND that recruitment to the qualifying training should be (a) through the Trainee grade, with secondment after a maximum of two years, or (b) by direct recruitment to the training course.**

225. The difference in recruitment methods should not affect the status of the Trainees. Those entering the Trainee grade prior to secondment would be working full-time during the pre-secondment period; they should therefore be regarded primarily as employees with a 100% contribution to service. Once training began the seconded Trainee and the Trainee recruited direct to training would be in the same position and their learning needs should have priority over the needs of the service. During training the Trainee would spend 50% of his time on theoretical study and practical assignments. Even during the 50% of his time devoted to the job the Trainee would not be fully productive since he would be learning how to apply newly learned skills. **We therefore estimate that during training a Trainee would make a contribution to service equivalent to 25% of that of a Basic Care Worker. Even during the pre-secondment period we** *RECOMMEND* **that the learning needs of Trainees should be paramount.**

CURRENT TRAINING IN THE HEALTH AND SOCIAL SERVICES

226. Having considered the training which we thought a mental handicap residential care worker would need we went on to compare this with the training currently provided in the health and the social services.

Current Nurse Training

227. The main mental handicap residential care training has always been that provided for the specialist nurses since, for reasons touched on in Chapter 1, nurses have always been by far the largest group among the residential care staff. Nurses who care for mentally handicapped people can be divided into three categories:—

a.	Registered nurses (Three year training)	RNMS (Registered Nurse for the Mentally Subnormal) in England and Wales.
		RNMD (Registered Nurse for Mental Defectives) in Scotland.
b.	Enrolled nurses (Two year training)	SEN (MS) (State Enrolled Nurse for the Mentally Subnormal) in England and Wales.
		Enrolled Nurse in Scotland (The Roll in Scotland is not divided into parts).
c.	Nursing assistants or auxiliaries. (No formal training – but the majority have some form of in-service training)	

The RNMS/RNMD training currently requires 2–3 'O' levels or an entry test, although for general nursing, and increasingly for RNMS/RNMD nursing, schools are laying down higher entry requirements. For Enrolled nurses there is no statutory entry requirement other than "a good general education" but for most schools applicants are required to pass an entry test. The syllabus for RNMS training was changed in 1957 and again in 1970; for RNMD training the syllabus was changed in 1964 and a new curriculum is currently under discussion. These changes were made in recognition of the new attitudes to mental handicap; the revisions introduced a greater concentration on the social caring aspect of the nurse's role and reduced the clinical element. The syllabus for the SEN(MS), which had not been changed since it was introduced in 1964, has recently been revised.

The Briggs Report

228.   The nursing training structure outlined in the previous paragraph is, however, currently under discussion following the report of the Briggs Committee. The proposals of the Briggs Committee have not yet been implemented, but the report recommended a broadly based modular training which would include four main clinical areas: medical; surgical; mental handicap or mental illness; and community nursing.

Current Training in the Social Services

229.   There is no separate profession of mental handicap residential care workers in the social services and there is accordingly no special training for this group. The Central Council for Education and Training in Social Work (CCETSW), which is responsible for the training of groups of staff working in the social services, promotes a number of courses suitable for residential and day care staff working with mentally handicapped people. At present the majority of residential care staff in local authority homes for mentally handicapped people are unqualified, but authorities are working towards one of the strategies proposed by the Birch Working Party[38] ie a 50% qualified (CQSW or CSS) workforce by the mid 1980s. The most frequently held qualifications

84

other than nursing qualifications are the CRSW (the Certificate in Residential Social Work), held by 17% of Officers in Charge and 5% of Deputies, and the CRCCYP and SCRCCYP (the Certificate or Senior Certificate in the Residential Care of Children and Young People), held by 9% of Officers in Charge and 12% of Deputies (figures from the OPCS Survey, Table 16). The CRSW is a one year, full-time course for senior staff in local authority or voluntary homes for elderly, mentally ill and physically and mentally handicapped people. The CRCCYP is a one year course for staff who have experience of residential child care. The last awards of the CRSW, CRCCYP and SCRCCYP will be made in 1981 and the resources of these courses will be merged with training provision leading to award of either the Certificate of Qualification in Social Work (CQSW) or the Certificate in Social Service (CSS).

230.   The Certificate of Qualification in Social Work is the only current professional qualification for field social workers, and posts designated for qualified field social workers should be filled by CQSW holders or staff holding the social work qualifications which preceded the CQSW. Increasingly the CQSW is becoming recognised as the professional qualification for residential social workers also. All CQSW courses require full-time study and a number of different types of courses are recognised by CCETSW for the awards of this qualification:
   a.   Non-Graduate Courses.—These are normally of two years' duration and students must be at least twenty before starting the course. Candidates must be capable of academic work beyond 'A' level standard. For students under 25 there is a five 'O' level entry requirement but for students over 25 there is no formal educational entry requirement.*
   b.   Degree Courses.—There are a number of four year degree courses in the social sciences on which one option is recognised by CCETSW as leading to the award of the CQSW.
   c.   Graduate Courses.—These are either one or two years in length, depending on the relevance of the student's first degree.

A number of CQSW courses highlight special areas of study (including residential work) in both curriculum content and practice placements. The CQSW is not however intended to provide substantial specialist teaching and social workers who wish to undertake specialist study do so by taking a post-qualifying course.

231.   The Certificate in Social Service is a new form of training which was introduced (in pilot schemes) in October 1975; by the end of 1978 222 Certificates should have been awarded. The Certificate is intended for groups of social services staff other than social workers. It is a modular course lasting a minimum of 2 years in which staff are released from their jobs on day-release or block-release for periods of training. The entry requirement for candidates under 21 is 5 'O' levels or equivalent. The CSS is a framework of training which is jointly planned by employing authorities and colleges (working through a Joint Management Committee) and approved by CCETSW. The

---

*There are a small number of three year courses catering for students with special needs, eg those with domestic responsibilities.

course framework currently provides for 3 modules, plus "practice" experience gained in the student's existing job under the direction of a study supervisor. The first, common unit is on "the context in which social service is provided" (CCETSW Paper 9:1)[39]. The second unit is one of 4 standard options focussing on: children and adolescents; adults; the elderly; or communities. The third unit is a special option designed to give students "the knowledge and skill to carry out specific tasks within the social services". CCETSW requires that the common unit should include "some knowledge of: the development of the individual in the family and in the community; human needs and the extent to which they are met; the formulation and implementation of social policy, both nationally and locally; and social service provision including the contribution which each student makes to it in his job".

232.   We are aware of the criticisms which have been voiced about the CSS —notably that it does not allow of sufficient specialisation; that it cannot compare with CQSW since the entry standard is lower; and that its "status" in unclear. We believe that many of the criticisms of CSS are unjust. On the question of specialisation the CCETSW framework proposes a minimum of 240 hours study for special units but asserts that "many of them may need to be considerably longer to meet the training needs of certain staff". Our views on this problem, and on the question of full-time or part-time study are described in paras 242–243. The problem of the standing of the CSS derives from concern about such matters as: the lack of a rigidly imposed entry requirement, the relationship between the CSS and the CQSW which is unclear to many people, and the fact that the course does not prepare one group of workers to do one particular job or perform one particular role. Fundamentally, these problems are all related to the principle of CSS as a framework for training rather than a qualifying course for a profession. Some of the difficulties are being ironed out as it becomes clearer what sort of people are taking CSS and what effect this training will have on their careers. We believe that financial recognition for CSS holders is very important and we are particularly glad to note that the National Joint Council for Local Authorities' Administrative, Professional, Technical and Clerical Staff has now decided to include the CSS in the list of awards whose holders are entitled to a qualifications allowance. At the same time we hope that the discussions within the social services professions on the distinction between "residential social work" and "residential care" will lead shortly to a clear definition of the two tasks, so that the CCETSW concept of the CQSW and the CSS as two distinct first line qualifications for these two distinct tasks will be clarified. Perhaps the most important problem facing the CSS at the moment however is the difficulty which faces any new training course: that of establishing itself. We believe that the "status" of a training derives mainly from the job for which it qualifies the trainee and that on this basis the CSS will soon become established as a valuable addition to the field of staff training.

THE TRAINING BODY

233.   Having decided that all mental handicap residential care staff should receive a common training we had to consider who should be responsible for this training. There appeared to be 4 possibilities:

(a) Responsibility shared between the General Nursing Councils (GNCs) and CCETSW.

(b) The GNCs to have overall responsibility.

(c) A new mental handicap residential care training body.

(d) CCETSW to have overall responsibility.

Shared Responsibility

234. *We rejected the first option of leaving training responsibilities conceptually and organisationally split as at present between the GNCs and CCETSW.* It seemed to us that the only certain way of ensuring that health and local authority mental handicap residential care staff received the same training was to train them together under the auspices of one training organisation. Nevertheless we recognised that the GNCs and CCETSW have a wealth of expertise in the training of staff and we did not wish this expertise to be lost.

The General Nursing Councils

235. The second possibility, of giving the GNCs responsibility for training both local authority mental handicap residential care staff and nurses had certain advantages. Schools of nursing currently provide by far the greater part of the specialist mental handicap residential care training and the nurse tutors make up the majority of the teaching staff with experience in this area. The GNC for England and Wales told us that they would be willing to continue to train nurses to provide residential care. The GNC for Scotland, on the other hand, told us that they did not regard themselves as a suitable body to train residential care staff.

236. In studying the mental handicap nurse training syllabuses we found that they provided considerable scope for emphasis on the social caring aspects of the nurse's role. We were, however, told (both in evidence and on visits) that the syllabus for Registered nurses is so long that schools of nursing cannot cover all the elements in depth and have to choose which subjects to emphasise. This choice helps to determine the attitudes of the staff who are being trained (although of course other factors, including ward practices, also help to mould staff attitudes). The survey conducted for us by OPCS also provided some information on this subject. Table 100 of the survey shows that, of Registered nurses trained since 1970 (ie since the most recent revision of the syllabus in England and Wales) and students still in training, nearly 75% thought that their training should place more emphasis on areas falling within the social caring side of their work (eg educational and training activities; ways of helping residents to develop emotionally and psychologically; ways of providing a homelike atmosphere for the residents; games and activities to do with the residents). For Enrolled nurses and pupils in training the corresponding figure was just under 50%. In general, the survey shows that the Registered nurses were more optimistic about the possibility of developing the potential of mentally handicapped people than were the Enrolled nurses and nursing assistants. (The fact that in any ward it is the junior staff who predominate therefore has important implications for staff training.) All of these facts suggested to us that despite the changes which have been made in the syllabuses, the training currently provided for mental handicap nurses has serious shortcomings of which nurses are aware.

237. We had, however, to consider not only the current training for nurses but also the proposals for restructuring this training. If the training system proposed by the Briggs Committee were implemented as it stands all nurses would take a common 18 months' initial training, much of which would be irrelevant to mental handicap residential care. Only those with the ability and desire for further training would then be able to go on to a more specialised course. *Thus nurses trained according to the Briggs proposals would have a much less specialist training than current nurses.* In the field of mental handicap the pattern proposed by the Briggs Committee would put the clock back to the time when the mental handicap nursing syllabus was a close copy of that for general nursing. We believe that this would be completely unacceptable to mental handicap nurses. *It would be impossible to prepare nurses adequately to operate our model of care within the pattern proposed by the Briggs Committee.* Even if a high degree of specialisation in mental handicap residential care could be provided post-Certificate the mental handicap nurses would inevitably form a small part of an organisation whose common denominator—training for the clinical nursing role—would be precisely that element which we believe to be over-emphasised in current mental handicap nurse training. This would still be true if the GNCs were to train local authority staff as well as nurses. A reliance on post-Certificate specialisation would in any case leave the nurses who do not progress beyond the first 18 months' training (ie those who are most in contact with the residents), without sufficient training for their residential caring rôle. *It was thus clear to us that, whether or not the Briggs Committee's proposals were implemented, nurse training could not provide a basis for training mental handicap residential care staff.*

A New Body

238. A completely new training body concerned solely with mental handicap care staff seemed at first sight an attractive proposition. A new training body would be able to respond quickly to changes in emphasis in mental handicap care and could offer courses tailored to the needs of one group of staff, rather than multi-client courses in which specialisms were available only as options. But a separate training council would mean that the training for mental handicap residential care would not be integrated with training for the residential care of other client groups. It is part of our philosophy that mentally handicapped people need to be thought of positively, in terms of the needs they have in common with the rest of us. Mental handicap residential care workers therefore need to learn first of all how to care for people, and then how to care for mentally handicapped people. *A separate training council would perpetuate the dogma of special services and special staff, reinforcing the isolation of mental handicap residential care.* Another factor is that mental handicap residential care staff are a comparatively small group; a separate qualification from a small training council would therefore lack the status of the more widely based qualifications in, for example, nursing and social work. The establishment of an independent, narrowly focused training system would go against the current thinking in staff training. It is now being recognised that staff who are doing a demanding job need to be able to move, after a period of years, to work with different clients or in a different setting; a separate council would make this sort of movement difficult.

The Central Council For Education And Training In Social Work

239.   The fourth option was to give CCETSW the responsibility for all mental handicap residential care staff training. In considering the training needs of mental handicap residential care staff we observed that many of these needs were common to all residential care staff training and it therefore seemed sensible to train all types of residential care staff within a common framework. The sort of training required by our model of care seemed to us to fit more appropriately in a social service training organisation than in a nurse training organisation. A common residential care training would broaden the horizons of all the staff involved and for mental handicap staff would provide the important input of training and experience in the care of normal adults and children. Too often in the past the potential of mentally handicapped people has not been recognised because staff training has focussed on the limiting aspects of mental handicap. An understanding of the normal growth and development of children and adults would help mental handicap residential care staff to understand what it is reasonable to expect of a normal individual or a physically or mentally handicapped person. The importance of shifting the emphasis from the handicap-centred approach to the individual-centred approach should not be underestimated. A common training framework for all residential care staff would also open the whole of the residential care service to mental handicap residential care workers and the senior advisory posts for residential services or mental handicap services would also be open to them.

240.   On the other hand we recognise that a very special drive will be needed to provide a new training which will:

a.   be acceptable to nurses as a new and appropriate alternative to the established and honourable profession to which they belong at present;

b.   ensure that residential care staff are fully prepared through long and intensive special elements in training to meet the wide range of special as well as general needs of mentally handicapped people, including the needs of those who are most profoundly handicapped, and

c.   be supported by the financial and human resources which are essential in order to bring about the major changes which will be required.

This second group of considerations led the Committee to reconsider very carefully the possibility of establishing a new training council which would act as the agent of change and lead the way in developing a new professionalism in the residential care of mentally handicapped people. We have already recognised, however, the significant dangers inherent in such a course, particularly that both the staff and the people they care for would be increasingly isolated from the community to which they belong. The proposal for a separate training council does not meet our requirement for a training which lies in the mainstream of residential care, and this would remain true, though to a lesser degree, even if the new council were to be seen as an interim arrangement designed to carry out the specific task of creating the new drive in training and, once this function had been fulfilled, to hand on its responsibility to CCETSW as the body responsible for training for all other forms of residential care. *In the absence of a solution which would meet all our criteria a significant body of opinion within the Committee held that despite these disadvantages a new council, on an interim basis, offered the best hope of providing the thrust for a major reorientation of the training effort.*

241. There is, however, one solution which provides the answer to all the problems we have canvassed, and which we therefore *RECOMMEND**: this is that the training of mental handicap residential care staff should be placed within the mainstream of residential care, under the aegis of CCETSW and following the broad framework of the Certificate in Social Service, but with the following additional provisions, all of which we regard as essential:

a. Special resources must be provided at the level necessary to ensure that all recruits are properly equipped to carry out the demanding tasks we have described.

b. A special group should be set up within CCETSW and maintained for as long as need be with the responsibility for designing special modules of training, ensuring that sufficient courses are set up which fully meet our requirements as to length and intensity of training, and ensuring that all that is best in nursing at present is retained and enhanced in the new model of training.

c. This group should have an operational arm—special Social Work Education Advisers whose task would be to promote the drive for change at local level.

THE CERTIFICATE IN SOCIAL SERVICE

242. Having accepted CCETSW as the most appropriate training body we did not feel bound to accept any of the existing trainings, if these should prove unsuitable. In paras 229–232 we described the two main arms of CCETSW training—the CSS and the CQSW. We considered both these types of training in relation to the needs of the residential care staff and our own model training programme. *The CSS, with its modular design is ideally suited to our concept of a two-part generic and specialist course.* The generic residential care component would be provided in the common and standard units while the special mental handicap teaching would be given in the special unit. Students would of course be supplementing the theoretical work with practice placements—the majority (though not all) of which would be in mental handicap establishments. To provide the detailed, in-depth study and practice in mental handicap residential care which we consider essential the special unit would need to be of at least 12 months. Although CCETSW recommends that "it should normally be possible for students to complete the three units in two years or a little longer" we could not see that a course lasting up to three years would present insuperable difficulties.

243. We have recommended two methods of recruitment for Trainees, with each Trainee undertaking a number of practice placements away from his own job. At present the CSS student is an employee throughout the course: "Although students may spend much of their time in one specific job, employers will be encouraged to provide a variety of work experience to extend the student's learning".[40] Under our proposals a Trainee would have a job of his own but would spend a number of placements in different

---

*Three members dissented from the majority view—see pages 150-160

locations—including homes and units for non-mentally handicapped people. There would thus be a greater need for colleges and employing authorities to plan together. While on a placement the Trainee would still be expected to do a job, just as if he were an employee.

244. We do not wish to make recommendations about the precise arrangements for a mental handicap residential care training within the CSS framework. If the units of study remain as at present a Trainee intending to work in the residential care of mentally handicapped children would take: the common unit; the standard unit on children and adolescents; and the special unit on mental handicap. Practice experience would be gained in the Trainee's own job, in a variety of residential Units for children and perhaps also in a residential or day special school or an observation and assessment centre. But the CSS is still in its infancy and the choice of standard units might be increased or the course might be altered in other ways in the light of experience. **We do however** *RECOMMEND* **that the CSS certificates should state clearly the specialism studied.** Those who had taken the mental handicap residential care CSS would then be able to use their certificate as evidence that they had undertaken the only training specifically provided for mental handicap residential care staff; similarly employers would know from the certificate whether or not an applicant was suitably qualified for a particular job. We understand that CSS certificates do include a reference to the units taken.

THE CERTIFICATE OF QUALIFICATION IN SOCIAL WORK

245. We explained in para 230 that the CQSW does not provide a substantial specialist training and does not prepare students specifically to work with particular client groups; it would not therefore be possible to incorporate our training proposals into the CQSW. Nevertheless the number of CQSW courses offering residential work as a "special area", with practice experience in residential settings is increasing. It may be expected in future that employers will designate certain posts in residential establishments as appropriate to be held by social workers and some CQSW holders who trained on courses giving special emphasis to residential work may wish to work in the field of mental handicap residential care. **But we** *RECOMMEND* **that CQSW trained staff who wish to work in the residential care of mentally handicapped people should have had specialist training equivalent to the mental handicap special unit on CSS.**

THE PROPOSED SYSTEM

246. We have said that we wish to encourage the development of a residential care profession. In the future, residential care staff in the social services will take the CSS or the CQSW as their training; clearly there would be advantages for mental handicap training in becoming part of this system. In paras 219–222 we described our recommended qualifying training: the CSS with modifications could provide this training. **We therefore** *RECOMMEND* **that CCETSW should make the necessary modifications and that the CSS should become the training for qualified mental handicap residential care staff.** Figure 16 shows how the proposed system would operate, with conversion

courses for staff entering from different disciplines and staff who had not taken the appropriate modules.

Practice Placements

247.   Under present arrangements CCETSW does not inspect practice placements when validating a course. It is for the Joint Management Committee, in the case of the CSS, and the college, in the case of the CQSW, to ensure that the experience supplied by a practice placement will be adequate. The GNCs on the other hand inspect all aspects of proposed practice placements outside the nurse training school before approving their use in whole or in part for a nurse training programme. The nurse training schools have experienced difficulty in finding placements outside hospitals and the GNCs currently have to accept placements which are not always the most suitable practice locations for mental handicap nurse training. This difficulty would be exacerbated by the proposed increase in the number of Trainees (see Chapter 4). Our model of care is based on small group living, ideally in small independent Units, but also in semi-autonomous wards and reorganised large and unhomelike buildings. Clearly there would be little point in sending all Trainees on practice placements to the few existing small Units—even if this were possible—since all practice experience would then bear no relation to the majority of work experience. But on the other hand Trainees should not gain practice experience in Units where they would be unable to learn how the social caring approach can be put into effect. **We** *RECOMMEND* **that all Trainees should have experience of small group living in some shape or form.** We believe that it should be possible to achieve this since many hospitals are already trying to increase ward autonomy. If practice placements were carefully chosen, so that the experience gained was both realistic and appropriate to the model of care, the Trainee would gain a balanced picture of the way in which theory can be put into effect. *To this end the special group within CCETSW should establish criteria to be used as guidance by local course planners for the selection of practice locations.*

248.   There is the additional problem that mentally handicapped people in residential accommodation are not evenly distributed throughout the country but are concentrated in a number of large hospitals. This would make it difficult for course planners to find sufficient placements within a reasonable travelling distance of the college. This maldistribution is also reflected in the comparatively small number of mentally handicapped people who are in residential care in the community. The mental handicap residential care Trainees would of course require experience not only in mental handicap hospitals and homes but also in children's and old people's homes, homes for physically handicapped people, and day centres—including ATCs, special schools and assessment centres. Placements and/or work experience have been gained in many of these locations by students on CSS and CQSW courses in the past, but course planners would need to build on this experience to increase both the number and scope of placements. **We therefore** *RECOMMEND* **that the special group within CCETSW should consider the problem of the effects of the maldistribution of mental handicap residential care establishments on the provision of practice placements and issue advice on the subject to course planners.**

FIGURE 16 – MODEL TRAINING STRUCTURE

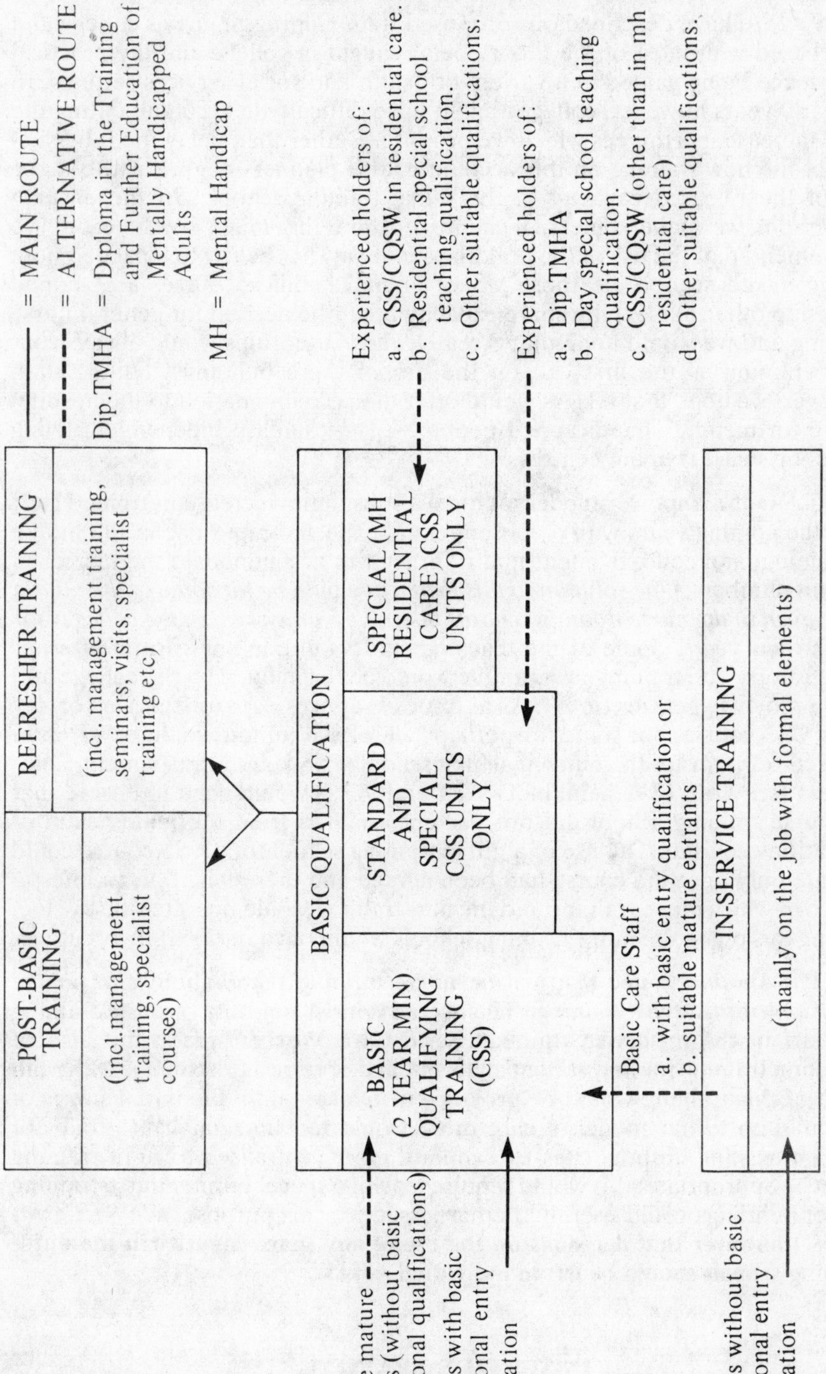

——— = MAIN ROUTE

– – – = ALTERNATIVE ROUTE

Dip.TMHA = Diploma in the Training and Further Education of Mentally Handicapped Adults

MH = Mental Handicap

POST-BASIC TRAINING	REFRESHER TRAINING
(incl. management training, specialist courses)	(incl. management training, seminars, visits, specialist training etc)

BASIC QUALIFICATION

BASIC (2 YEAR MIN) QUALIFYING TRAINING (CSS)	STANDARD AND SPECIAL CSS UNITS ONLY	SPECIAL (MH RESIDENTIAL CARE) CSS UNITS ONLY

Basic Care Staff
a. with basic entry qualification or
b. suitable mature entrants

IN-SERVICE TRAINING

(mainly on the job with formal elements)

Experienced holders of:
a. CSS/CQSW in residential care.
b. Residential special school teaching qualification.
c. Other suitable qualifications.

Experienced holders of:
a. Dip.TMHA
b. Day special school teaching qualification.
c. CSS/CQSW (other than in mh residential care)
d. Other suitable qualifications.

Suitable mature entrants (without basic educational qualifications)

Entrants with basic educational entry qualification

Entrants without basic educational entry qualification

The Nurse Training Schools

249.   We have described our proposed training programme as college and Unit based with most of the theory being taught in college and the practical experience being gained in a variety of health and social services settings. In the early years however, colleges might have difficulty in accommodating the large increase in Trainees which we propose. Rather than delay the introduction of the new training on this account course planners might wish to make use of the released capacity in the nurse training schools. In the ensuing paragraphs we make some suggestions on how this might be done but we recommend that the use of the building should always be left to local decision. In the mixed schools (ie those where mental handicap nurses are trained alongside other nurses) the spare capacity might be needed for general nurse training and we would hope that Area Health Authorities would always consider training as the first call on the use of these buildings. Failing that, however, we hope that AHAs would offer the accommodation to the hospital to use for mentally handicapped people—eg to establish independent living Units, or social training centres.

250.   Our manpower model requires a substantial increase in trained staff over the coming years with a consequential expected rapid rise in the intake to training, and colleges might find it difficult to accommodate the increased student numbers. *One solution to this problem would be for some of the tuition to be given in the nurse training schools instead of, or as well as, the colleges for the first few years.* Some of the teaching staff would, in any case, be former nurse tutors. The training programme would be formulated by the college and the employing agencies (ie AHAs and social services departments) as for any other CSS course, but some, or perhaps all, of the tuition would be given in the lecture rooms of the nurse teaching school. CSS Joint Management Committees (see CCETSW pamphlets 9.2[40] and 9.3[41]) would need to ensure that the nurse training school did not become isolated from the mainstream of education provision.The use of a nurse training school for a CSS course could operate only once the course had been agreed and there might be an interim period in which nurse training and the new training would operate side by side. During this phase the nurse training schools would of course be fully occupied.

251.   *Another major use for the nurse training schools might be in the provision of in-service training.* This would consist not only of basic training for staff in the in-service trained (Basic Care Worker) grade but also of induction training for new staff at all levels, and of refresher training. Although much of this training would be provided at Unit level, in the initial stages of the build-up to our model of care there would remain significant groups of staff on existing hospital sites for whom a more centralised form of training might be appropriate; this would require teaching space. Former nurse training school buildings could usefully be harnessed for this purpose. We *RECOMMEND* **however that decisions on the use of any spare capacity in the nurse training schools should be left to individual AHAs.**

IN-SERVICE TRAINING

252.   Apart from the qualifying training which we have recommended, staff at all levels also need in-service training. This should be of three types:

a.   induction training for new staff at all levels;

b.   refresher training—including formal courses on management, or new techniques etc and informal group discussions; and

c.   basic training for Basic Care Staff.

We *RECOMMEND* **that employing authorities should designate a training organiser or some other person to ensure that each member of staff is involved in an on-going training programme suited to his needs.**The training organiser should have appropriate preparation (ie training) for his duties. In a large authority these duties would probably warrant a full-time appointment; in other cases the post of training organiser might be combined with some other administrative or professional job. The training organiser's role would not be limited to in-service training, he should also liaise with training bodies to ensure that local in-service and national statutory courses complemented rather than duplicated each other.

Induction Training

253.   *The training organiser should ensure that each new member of staff receives formal induction training within a reasonable time of starting work.* This induction training should include:

a.   Instruction on the aims and working methods of the Unit.

b.   Details of the support available to the Unit staff from social work, nursing, medical and other services.

c.   Information on the organisation and management hierarchy of the employing authority, including advice on how to make complaints and where and how to seek advice.

The first of these three subjects would probably need to be taught within the Unit itself but the other two could be provided centrally by the authority. The factual instruction involved might be given by the training organiser himself, but the induction training should also include visits to appropriate Units and offices and talks from staff of the authority.

Refresher Training

254.   *Both Basic and qualified residential care staff need refresher training throughout their careers.* Some staff will need preparation for management or other new responsibilities, most will occasionally need to learn new skills or refresh old ones, and all staff will need to widen their horizons periodically—by discussing new ideas on mental handicap residential care, visiting other units and relating their experience to current policies. Refresher courses should also be the means of encouraging people to return to mental handicap residential care after a break of some years—eg to raise a family. The training organiser should ensure that those staff who need formal training (eg a management or post-basic training course) whether on a nationally recognised course promoted by a training body, or on a course run by the employing authority, are released for training at the appropriate time. He should also organise the informal refresher training, with seminars, lectures, visits etc at regular intervals. The training organiser should help to build up a positive attitude towards training in his authority and should respond to training demands from both junior staff and managers. **We** *RECOMMEND* **that every member of staff**

should receive formal induction training and should be encouraged to attend refresher or specialist training courses.

Training for Basic Care Staff

255.   Our model of care depends upon a Basic Care Worker grade in which the staff have been taught the fundamental principles of the residential care of mentally handicapped people. *Nursing and care assistants have in the past suffered from the lack of a comprehensive and well planned training scheme, yet these staff are direct residential care workers, constantly in touch with the residents.* The abilities and attitudes of Basic Care Staff have a profound effect on the life-style of the residents; we therefore attach particular importance to the training provided for these people. We envisage this training as predominantly on-the-job tuition, given by personal advice and guidance from the senior staff of the Unit, but it should also include a significant formal element. Senior staff, up to and including the Head of the Unit, should regard the training of junior staff as an integral part of their job; our manpower recommendations take account of the time which senior staff should devote to staff training. The formal element of the in-service training should include such components as lectures, visits, seminars, films and self-teaching packs, and might include some college-based tuition. We recommend that there should be a nationally agreed minimum time allocated to this training. The Report of the Working Party on Manpower and Training for the Social Services[38] recommended the provision of in-service training for all staff equivalent to two weeks in each year. We regard this as the minimum for all staff and would expect the training for the Basic Care Staff to require rather more time than this, particularly in the early years of an employee's career. This in-service training should be regarded as standing in its own right and should not either be a prerequisite for qualifying training or confer exemption from such training. The syllabus for this training should include: basic hygiene; emergency procedures; incontinence; feeding; toiletting etc; home safety; information on normal behaviour and variations in behaviour of mentally handicapped people; and basic activities of daily living, including matters applicable to general residential care. We *RECOMMEND* that employing authorities should provide formal in-service training of at least 2 weeks equivalent in each year for all Basic Care Staff.

256.   Our recommendations on training for Basic Care Staff involve not only a considerable increase in the time devoted to such training but also a new attitude to these staff. Both the Basic Care Staff and those who supervise them will have to rethink their approach to training and responsibility. Some staff might find this difficult and employing authorities should ensure that the reasons for the increase in training and the benefits to be expected from it are carefully explained to all staff. In small Units it might be difficult to release staff for training but this should be covered by our proposed increase in staff numbers. *We urge employing authorities not to regard this part of our package as expendable; a well-trained Basic Care Worker grade is integral to our model of care.*

NURSING CARE FOR SICK MENTALLY HANDICAPPED PEOPLE

257.   We have recommended that mental handicap residential care should be given by residential care staff, whatever the location. These staff would be

the major element of the caring team, assisted by other specialists such as nurses, psychiatrists etc. It is part of our philosophy of care that mentally handicapped people should use general social and public services wherever possible. This means that when mentally handicapped people require hospital treatment they should be looked after in the ordinary way by general or sick children's nurses. At present when mentally handicapped people are admitted to a general hospital they are frequently accompanied by a mental handicap nurse, at the request of the general hospital whose nurses "could not cope" with a mentally handicapped patient. Such patients are usually discharged sooner than other patients, since the general hospital staff know that the patient will return to a "hospital" where he will be looked after by "nurses". When all mental handicap Units are staffed by residential care staff this will no longer be the case, and the general hospitals will have to retain mentally handicapped patients for as long as any other patients. We believe that the general or sick children's nurse should be able to cope with all types of patient; if however the hospital requires assistance with a mentally handicapped patient a member of the residential care staff from the patient's home Unit could accompany him during his hospital stay. This should also apply to mentally handicapped people requiring psychiatric hospital treatment. In addition mentally handicapped children who have to be admitted to hospital have the same emotional needs as other children and if the child's parents are unable to provide emotional support—by visiting and staying overnight—the residential care staff from the home unit should take on this role. **We therefore *RECOMMEND* that mentally handicapped people who require general, paediatric, or psychiatric hospital treatment should be cared for in hospital by general, sick children's or psychiatric nurses and that the training of these nurses should include an understanding of mental handicap.**

SEVERELY MENTALLY AND MULTIPLY HANDICAPPED PEOPLE

258.   In our model of care we have reluctantly recognised that some mentally handicapped people could not be cared for in the ordinary small living Units (including small living Units in large hospitals) which we propose. Certain mentally handicapped people have a temporary or permanent need for specialised skills because of the nature of their handicap. Some of these people will have severe and intractable forms of socially unacceptable behaviour, others may have specific long-term disabilities such as sensory deficits which call for special skills in the staff who care for them. All should be cared for in the same way as other mentally handicapped people. These severely mentally and multiply handicapped people will need the help of residential care staff and general, psychiatric or sick children's nurses with specialised skills, plus the resources of an inter-disciplinary back-up team for as long as their special requirements persist. *Working with only the most difficult cases presents a particular set of problems for staff and these problems can best be resolved by creating a pool of staff who gain continuous experience with the most difficult residents and who share their problems and learn from each other.* Both the qualified residential care staff and the nurses working with these people would require post-qualifying training. For the qualified residential care staff this should cover: behaviour modification; care of adults or children with specific types of mental handicap; and assessment and observation of

multiple handicaps. (Basic Care Staff would also be needed in the short stay Units but we do not recommend any additional training for them.) The nurses would require post-qualifying training to enable them to apply their nursing skills to profoundly mentally and multiply handicapped people.**We *RECOMMEND* that the General Nursing Councils and the Central Council for Education and Training in Social Work should collaborate on the development of post-qualifying courses for general, psychiatric and sick children's nurses and residential care staff working with very severely handicapped residents.**

POST-QUALIFYING TRAINING

259.   Post-qualifying training should help qualified residential care staff to learn and to develop particular skills and techniques (eg management skills and behaviour modification techniques), to deepen their knowledge of mental handicap, to refresh knowledge and skills acquired earlier and to increase their awareness of the wider context of mental handicap residential care (through knowledge of the health and personal social services framework). Courses should be provided by educational establishments and validated by CCETSW. Some courses might be of a few weeks duration, concentrating on a particular problem in detail, while others might last up to a year, dealing with more complex themes. **We *RECOMMEND* that post-qualifying courses should be available for all staff at the Qualified Care Worker grade and above.**

THE TRAINING STAFF

260.   At present mental handicap nurse training is conducted by nurse tutors in schools of nursing, while social services training is the responsibility of lecturers in educational establishments. Both organisations bring in staff from different disciplines to teach specific subjects. Our proposed qualifying training requires tutors based in Colleges of Further Education and practice supervisors based in employing agencies. The college tutorial staff should comprise a balance of experienced mental handicap residential care staff and "pure" academics; the practice supervisors should be experienced residential care workers.

261.   Future training staff (tutors and practice supervisors) will need special training: experienced residential care staff will need to learn teaching techniques and academic staff will need to learn about the residential care of mentally handicapped people. The Advisory Committee on the Supply and Training of Teachers has recommended that all untrained new entrants to full-time teaching in further education should undertake a systematic induction training course, normally during their first year of teaching.[42] This training course should amount to no less than 50 days of training. Induction training of this type would be appropriate for tutors and supervisors lacking teaching qualifications or experience and our proposed CSS special unit could provide the necessary background in mental handicap residential care for academic staff lacking experience in this area.

Nurse Tutors

262.   There are currently 3 types of nurse tutor:
   (a)   Registered Nurse Tutors (RNTs)—these are in the main Registered nurses who have completed a 2 year university or polytechnic course.

RNTs teaching mental handicap learners may not always be RNMS/RNMD.

(b) Clinical nurse teachers—these are Registered nurses who have completed a 3–6 month course, who act as "study supervisors" but may also lecture in the nurse training school. Those who teach mental handicap learners are usually RNMS/RNMD.

(c) Unqualified nurse tutors—these are senior RNMS/RNMD nurses who, because of the shortage of RNTs, act as tutors.

There will be a pressing need for teaching staff and practice supervisors on the new mental handicap residential care qualifying training. *There are of course some existing CSS courses which include mental handicap and/or residential care components; the tutors and practice supervisors on these courses will have an important role to play in helping to devise and man the new courses. But the nurse teaching staff will provide a reservoir of staff with experience of both mental handicap and teaching techniques. With appropriate conversion training the nurse tutors and clinical teachers should provide the backbone of the new tutorial and supervisory staff.*

263.   Some RNTs are qualified teachers and it should be relatively easy for them to transfer from health authority to education authority employment. Some unqualified nurse tutors also possess teaching qualifications and they too should have no difficulties in transferring. **We strongly** *RECOMMEND* **that health and education authorities jointly consider the question of transferability of teaching qualifications so that the resources of nurse teaching staff can be used to best advantage in the new training.** The clinical nurse teachers might opt to become practice supervisors, a role where their combination of practical and teaching experience would be very valuable. The qualifying training is not the only mental handicap residential care staff training we are recommending and teaching staff will also be required in the training for Basic Care Staff and the various other forms of in-service training. We hope that some of the existing nurse teaching staff will choose to become involved in these important elements of our training model.

Preliminary Training for Tutors and Supervisors

264.   Those who will become tutors and practice supervisors on our proposed CSS scheme will need special preparation for their new roles. We understand that some CSS schemes include a preliminary course on which tutors and supervisors learn about the concept of the CSS. Tutors and practice supervisors will play an important role in ensuring that our model of care is conveyed to Trainees; if the teaching staff do not fully understand or are not in sympathy with our model there is little hope of its being introduced. **We therefore** *RECOMMEND* **that all our new mental handicap residential care CSS schemes should include preliminary courses for staff and that these courses should be extended to include instruction in our model of care.** For existing nurse teaching staff these preliminary courses would serve as conversion

training and would include an explanation of how the new training and the new concepts of care differ from existing theory and practice.

NURSE TRAINING IN THE SPECIAL HOSPITALS

265. Special Hospitals provide residential care for persons detained under the Mental Health Act 1959 who require special security on account of their dangerous, violent or criminal propensities. People who meet this criteria and who are suffering from mental handicap or severe mental handicap are normally admitted to either Rampton or Moss Side hospitals. Each of these hospitals has a mental handicap nurse training school. In the light of our training recommendations the Department of Health and Social Security will need to look urgently at the future training needs of the staff in these hospitals. This review will be complicated by the fact that many of the patients in both hospitals suffer from mental illness as well as mental handicap, and over the years, because of the overcrowding at Broadmoor, there has been a tendency by the Department to admit more persons suffering solely from mental illness or psychopathic disorder into Rampton or Moss Side.

CO-ORDINATION PROBLEMS

266. A major feature of our proposed form of training is that it involves not just a new syllabus or a new format of training but, for the majority of staff, a new training body. There would be considerable problems of co-ordination in gradually winding down the existing GNC courses while at the same time building up new courses within the CCETSW framework. The General Nursing Councils of Scotland and England and Wales have built up a substantial body of knowledge and expertise in training staff to work in mental handicap residential care. *The special group within CCETSW would undoubtedly wish to call on the experiences of those who have been devising and implementing the current training courses in addition to drawing on other disciplines for advice and assistance in devising the new courses.* The special group would need to work up a programme for the implementation of our recommendations within the CCETSW framework and to undertake the detailed work which would be needed before a CSS special unit on mental handicap residential care could be introduced.

267. Since the new training requires joint action by colleges and employing authorities its introduction would require co-ordination at a local as well as a national level. Social services departments will have had experience in planning courses jointly with colleges but for NHS authorities this would be a relatively new activity; liaison would be required so that joint approaches could be made to colleges. This liaison would raise difficult problems which would need to be resolved locally and arrangements for planning courses would need to be flexible enough to meet local conditions. **We therefore** *RECOMMEND* **that health, social services and education authorities should come together in local committees to plan the introduction of the new training.** These committees would seek their own solutions to local problems but would look to the special group within CCETSW for advice on policy issues of national importance.

100

A FINAL DATE FOR THE CHANGEOVER

268. We believe that agreement on the final date for the award of the GNC qualifications in mental handicap nursing should be left to the GNCs and CCETSW. The three bodies would need to establish how soon the new training could be got underway before the GNCs could put a date to the ending of their training; the implementation of the Briggs proposals would also have a bearing on the decision. *We are however convinced that for the sake of the staff involved and for those thinking of taking up mental handicap nursing a final date should be decided on and announced as quickly as possible.* We mention in Chapter 6 the need to safeguard the status of nursing qualifications during the interim period and after the new qualification has been introduced.

THE MECHANISMS OF CHANGE

269. In considering training for mental handicap residential care staff we had to think not only of the new recruits but also of the system in which they would be working and the existing staff who made up that system. We have heard complaints from both nurses and social services staff that they are frequently unable to apply what they have been taught in training to their work on the Unit. In the case of nurses it is partly because the physical environment of a large old hospital makes it difficult, if not impossible, to create the homelike atmosphere which they have been taught is desirable and partly—and this applies also to the social services—because staffing levels often do not permit enlightened practices to be carried out. For a prolonged period in the past, services for mentally handicapped people were starved of resources. Over the past 10 years the picture has begun to change and positive efforts have been made to redress the balance, but in both the health and social services there is still a long way to go. The 1971 White Paper proposed a programme which would take 20 years to achieve and even then a considerable number of large old hospitals would still be in use. In recommending a new approach to training we have had to recognise the probability that unless the money is found for radical changes many old and unsuitable buildings will still be there for the foreseeable future. Our remit does not permit us to make recommendations about services as opposed to staffing, but the two are inextricably intertwined. *It is clear to us that if our model of care is to be brought into effect the mental handicap services must be allocated an increasing share of resources.*

270. The problems associated with introducing our new form of training are not simply problems of finance and resources. We also have to overcome the initial reaction against change which is intrinsic to any large organisation. In both nursing and the social services traditions have been built up over the years and many staff would find it difficult to accept that these should be swept away. Staff who have been trained in or conditioned by the older less socially oriented models of care inevitably find it easier to run a large hospital as one Unit with centralised services and uniformly applied rules. In these circumstances the policies and practices taught in training can quickly be "unlearned" on the ward or in the Unit. Staff who have worked for years in a hierarchical and strongly centralised system may find it difficult to understand and encourage the new ideas in mental handicap residential care which the recent

Trainees have learned. There is thus a danger that any new emphasis in training could be dissipated by a lack of understanding of the reasons for the changes. This danger could be averted by ensuring that existing staff have a clear understanding of the reasons for and effects of the introduction of the new training. **We therefore** *RECOMMEND* **that all existing staff should attend seminars and study days to learn about our report and discuss its implications for them.** This activity should not be restricted to nurses and local authority residential care staff; it should be inter-disciplinary, involving all the professions with an interest in the treatment and care of mentally handicapped people. We think that staff would welcome the opportunity to attend these study days and to participate actively in bringing the new model of care into effect.

271.   It was suggested to us that the most cost-effective method of introducing the new form of training would be to start by re-training the officers in charge of Units. It is argued that the person in charge sets the tone for the whole establishment and could thus ensure that our new model of care was introduced quickly and easily. *We are sure that the heads of living Units must be the agents of change and that they will bear the main responsibility for altering the ideas and working methods of staff. Nevertheless we reject the idea of re-training the senior staff. They have had years of professional experience in caring for mentally handicapped people and do not need to start again from scratch.* What these staff do need is an understanding of the changes we propose. We hope that Heads of living Units will read our report thoughtfully; past experience has shown how vital it is that senior staff should be fully involved in the processes of change. **We** *RECOMMEND* **that employing authorities and training bodies should re-examine their existing courses for senior staff to ensure that, in the light of our Report, senior staff are given the opportunity to explore the new perspectives on mental handicap residential care.**

CHAPTER 6 – ORGANISATION AND MANAGEMENT

INTRODUCTION

272.   We started this report by looking at mentally handicapped people and their needs; in this Chapter we consider the ways in which client needs and staff needs can be put together in a workable organisation. First we look at the existing organisation of mental handicap residential care workers in the health and social services. Then we go on to explain the model which our recommendations require, based on factors such as the skill levels at which work should be performed, the career outlets for residential care staff, relationships between residential care staff and other professional groups, staff management and accountability, discipline, and representation at top levels of management.

EXISTING MANAGEMENT STRUCTURES

The NHS

273.   The career structure of mental handicap nurses is part of the general career structure for nurses in the NHS. Figures 17–19 show how, in theory, the ward nursing team fits into the management hierarchy. In practice the situation is likely to be rather different. Figures from our OPCS survey suggest that the average size of a mental handicap hospital ward is 30 beds for adults and 20 beds for children (OPCS Table 23). In an adult ward of 30 beds there would probably be 4 staff on duty in the daytime: a Charge Nurse, an Enrolled Nurse and 2 Nursing Assistants. A children's ward of 20 beds would most likely have 5 or 6 staff: a Charge Nurse, perhaps a Staff Nurse and an Enrolled Nurse and 2 Nursing Assistants (OPCS Tables 7 and 29). Some adults' and children's wards might have a student or pupil nurse on duty. A mental handicap hospital of 400 beds might have 8–10 Nursing Officers and one or two Senior Nursing Officers. The Divisional Nursing Officer for the psychiatric division would in most cases be responsible for both mental handicap and mental illness nursing and would be based at one of the psychiatric hospitals in the District. In theory a nurse on any part of the Register could, with additional management training, progress to the highest ranks in nursing. In practice an RNMS/RNMD nurse would be unlikely to proceed beyond Div NO unless she was also SRN/RGN and/or RMN. (Indeed the majority of Div NOs in the psychiatric divisions are Registered on more than one part of the Register). An Enrolled Nurse can progress no further than Senior Enrolled Nurse (a rare post which few Enrolled Nurses are likely to achieve).

The Social Services

274.   There is no specialist national career structure for the residential care staff employed by local authorities in homes for mentally handicapped people. The National Joint Council for Local Authority Administrative, Professional, Technical and Clerical Services lays down pay scales for Officers in Charge, based on the number and type of residents in the home. The same pay scales

FIGURE 17 – MENTAL HANDICAP NURSING CAREER STRUCTURE (ENGLAND, WALES AND SCOTLAND)

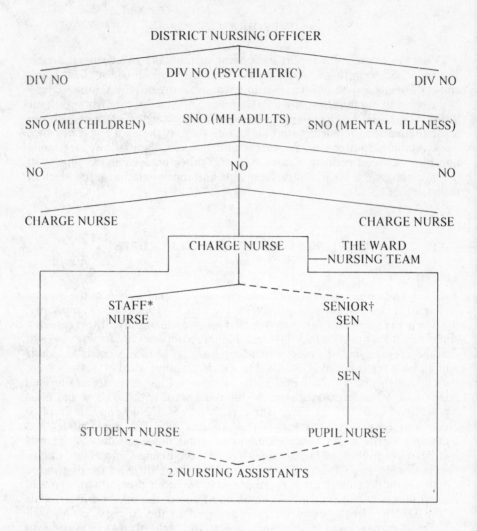

DISTRICT NURSING OFFICER

DIV NO   DIV NO (PSYCHIATRIC)   DIV NO

SNO (MH CHILDREN)   SNO (MH ADULTS)   SNO (MENTAL ILLNESS)

NO   NO   NO

CHARGE NURSE   CHARGE NURSE

CHARGE NURSE   THE WARD NURSING TEAM

STAFF* NURSE   SENIOR† SEN

SEN

STUDENT NURSE   PUPIL NURSE

2 NURSING ASSISTANTS

KEY

——— MANAGEMENT AND PROMOTION HIERARCHY

– – – = MANAGEMENT HIERARCHY ONLY

* = IF AVAILABLE

† = IF NO STAFF NURSE

DIV NO = DIVISIONAL NURSING OFFICER
SNO = SENIOR NURSING OFFICER
NO = NURSING OFFICER
MH = MENTALLY HANDICAPPED
SEN = STATE ENROLLED NURSE

FIGURE 18 – HIGHER NURSING STRUCTURE IN ENGLAND

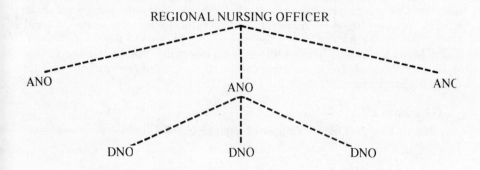

REGIONAL NURSING OFFICER

ANO

ANO

ANC

DNO

DNO

DNO

FIGURE 19: HIGHER NURSING STRUCTURE IN SCOTLAND AND WALES

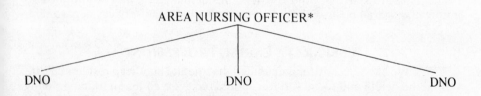

AREA NURSING OFFICER*

DNO

DNO

DNO

KEY

ANO = AREA NURSING OFFICER

DNO = DISTRICT NURSING OFFICER

* = CHIEF AREA NURSING OFFICER IN SCOTLAND

------- = PROMOTION HIERACHY PLUS MONITORING AND
CO-ORDINATING RELATIONSHIP

————— = PROMOTION HIERARCHY AND MANAGEMENT
RELATIONSHIP

Regional and Area Nursing Officers are supported by Regional and Area Nurses.

(for "Supervisory staff of residential accommodation provided under the National Assistance Act 1948 and Sections 6 and 8 of the Mental Health Act 1959") are to be used for "supporting staff", the exact grading being "at the discretion of the employing authority". Care assistants are paid on manual worker grades. There is, however, considerable uniformity between local authorities on the staffing of residential homes, despite the freedom allowed. Every home has a Warden or Officer in Charge and a number of supporting ·staff. The titles of the residential care staff vary between authorities; the following are some commonly used titles:

Officer in Charge/Warden

2nd in Charge/Deputy Officer in Charge

3rd in Charge

Group Leader/Assistant Officer in Charge

Care Assistant

There are no regulations about the employment of unqualified staff in residential care, and as our survey shows (OPCS Table 16) one third of Officers in Charge, half of Deputies, and four fifths of the other residential care staff have no formal qualifications in nursing or social work. Beyond the Officer in Charge level the career of a residential care worker in the social services is uncertain. Most authorities have a Homes Adviser with a non-managerial role in support of residential homes, and these posts would be open to experienced residential care staff. Beyond this level residential care staff would look to purely managerial posts within the local authority social services department.

A SEPARATE CARING PROFESSION?

275.   We have already recommended that mental handicap residential care staff in the health and social services should receive a common training. Many of the individuals and groups who submitted evidence to us went further and suggested the establishment of a separate mental handicap caring profession, or a separate mental handicap service. The Briggs Committee recommended that "a new caring profession for the mentally handicapped should emerge gradually". There has however been a wide range of opinion on what the Briggs Committee meant by "a new caring profession". The majority of those who gave evidence to us seemed to think of a new profession as a group of people trained in the residential care of mentally handicapped people only, with no outlet into careers with other client groups (without separate training), and with no admission into the group except at the basic level. Many people saw such a new caring profession as the nucleus for an independent service exclusively concerned with the treatment and care of mentally handicapped people; there are clear attractions in such an idea. With a separate profession standards of services for mentally handicapped people would be safeguarded by the special knowledge and skills of the staff. The staff would be well motivated since they had chosen to work with mentally handicapped people and their families and could be their advocates, pressing for more resources and improvements in services. Staff would be able to identify with a distinct professional group and gain the status which that implies, and existing nurses might be willing to accept such an alternative profession. There would be a

clearly defined promotion ladder which would not require staff to go outside mental handicap to gain promotion. Parents would have one service to turn to for all types of advice and help.

276.   But there is no precedent for establishing a profession based solely on a client group and it is unlikely that the new profession would in fact achieve "professional status". The numbers in the profession would be small, with few senior posts and would therefore not have a powerful voice at the policy making resource allocation level. An enclosed group could lead to even greater isolation of mentally handicapped people than already exists and could militate against other professions taking responsibility for them in the normal provision of services; this would be even more likely if the new profession were isolated in a separate new mental handicap service. The mobility which is currently possible within the various branches of nursing and within the social services would be lost since a special profession would tend to limit or stop entry at other than the basic level and to close the door on older entrants wishing to change career. The lack of many senior posts might make the profession unattractive to the more able candidates.

277.   Other interpretations of the Briggs Committee's recommendation have been that a new caring profession means a group of people, including not only residential care staff but also other staff such as teachers, who specialise in working with mentally handicapped people but retain their separate professional identity; or a group of people brought together by their training, who are residential care staff first but want to look after mentally handicapped people, and who would have the opportunity to work with other client groups if they so wished with only a minimum of retraining. Another view is that the Briggs Committee did not intend to recommend the creation of a new profession as such – which would, in any case, have been outside their terms of reference – but rather to take note of the practical effect of the 1971 White Paper policy of shifting the balance of care from hospitals to the community. The result of this policy would be a sizeable community-based profession of residential care workers, so that a "new profession" would emerge of its own accord.

278.   Having weighed up all the arguments we concluded that *the interests of mentally handicapped people would not be best served by the creation of a separate, new, specialist profession or a separate mental handicap service. Instead, as we have said in Chapter 5, we would prefer to see the development of a residential care profession within which there would be a variety of specialisms.* The training for this profession should be such as to enable staff to progress along a clear career path either within the chosen specialist field – such as mental handicap – or within the wider field of general residential care. **We therefore RECOMMEND that a separate new mental handicap residential caring profession should not be created;** mental handicap residential care staff should be part of the general residential care profession within which staff, could, after suitable training, practise a variety of specialisms.

A UNIFIED STRUCTURE

279.   *We do not believe that our concept of a profession of residential care staff, sharing a common framework of training and working in both the health*

and social services, could be achieved satisfactorily without a unified career structure; free movement between authorities and equality of opportunity could not be assured without a common hierarchy. We therefore had to consider what sort of structure was called for by our model of care.

280.   The organisation and management of residential care staff should provide the framework within which our model of care could most efficiently be brought into effect. The structure would thus need to be flexible enough to operate in a variety of living situations; it should maximise the opportunities for teamwork both within Units and across professional boundaries; it should allow for individual independence backed by professional support; above all it should be client focussed so that the Unit hierarchy is organised to meet the needs of the residents, and higher levels of management are organised to help the Unit staff to carry out their duties.

Levels of Work, Skill and Training

281.   As a first step we considered how many levels of work were required for the provision of residential care to mentally handicapped people. We tried not to confuse levels of work, levels of skill and levels of training since an individual may work at different skill levels on different aspects of one level of work. For the purposes of our structure we defined the level of work according to the task to be done; for example the task of taking a group of mentally handicapped people out for a walk would be at a lower level of *work* than the task of teaching an individual to feed, wash or dress himself. Levels of skill we defined as relating to the performance of the task, while we saw levels of training as relating to the training input required to improve the performance of staff. We have dealt with training in Chapter 5, here we are primarily concerned with levels of skill since we wish to see every care task exploited by skilled staff to provide the utmost benefit to the resident.

282.   Starting at Unit level we saw a broad division between those who have received a full, qualifying training and are looking to mental handicap residential care for a professional career and those who, being either unable or unwilling to undertake a demanding, qualifying training, are nonetheless able to offer service of a more practical kind. The latter we have called Basic Care Staff, the former Qualified Staff.

Basic Care Staff

283.   It was suggested to us that we should recommend the establishment of a 100% qualified profession, and that unqualified staff are currently employed largely because of a lack of qualified staff or for reasons of economy. We reject this argument and would prefer to retain the advantages of the present nursing and care assistant grades and to improve the training and status of these staff. The present assistants working in mental handicap often come into the service late, with no desire to progress up a career ladder. Since many of them are unable or unwilling to undertake full qualifying training they are not liable to be removed from the Unit at short notice for long training courses, or to move from Unit to Unit to gain experience and seek promotion. For these reasons the nursing and care assistants inject a vital element of stability into the Unit. In addition, since most of them live close to their place

of work they can bring ready-made links with the local community. The assistants are usually older than the student/pupil nurses and trainee residential care staff, and many will have brought up their own families; they can therefore bring to their work valuable maturity and experience.

284. We wish to preserve all these advantages of the assistant grades but also to add a compulsory formal training (see Chapter 5). *With careful selection, the training we recommend, and with support and guidance from their senior staff the Basic Care Staff can complement the work of the qualified staff in many of the tasks of residential care.* Basic Care Staff should perform the basic tasks of personal care, and assist in the teaching of social skills and the implementation of individual care programmes. Unqualified staff do not at present participate in assessment and case conferences (indeed the OPCS Report – Table 51 – shows that just over half of the *qualified* nursing staff do not participate in case conferences). We believe that Basic Care Staff will be able to make a valuable contribution to the design of future programmes through their observations and their close relationships with the residents. In these instances, as in all other spheres, Basic Care Staff and qualified staff will work as a team, bringing their own individual skills to the task in hand.

285. Although we refer in Chapter 5 to "qualifying" training we do not use the term "unqualified" to describe those who do not take this training. "Unqualified staff" may be a fair description of some current nursing and care assistants but it would not be appropriate for Basic Care Staff. *Because of the thorough in-service training which we are recommending for them, we refer to Basic Care Staff not as "unqualified staff" but as "in-service trained staff".* Although we have recommended minimum entry requirements for young people seeking qualifying training, these would not apply to suitable late entrants. There would therefore be nothing to prevent Basic Care Staff who were able to complete the qualifying training from progressing to the Trainee grade. Indeed school leavers of 16 and 17 might enter the service as Basic Care Staff until they were old enough (ie 18) to enter the Trainee grade.

Trainees

286. We *RECOMMEND* **that the qualifying training should start at the age of 18, since we do not wish to see anyone taking on the responsibilities of a qualified staff member before the age of 20.** Since Trainees will be training to become Qualified Care Staff (see para 287 below) much of their time would be spent assisting these staff, but they would also spend some time on Basic Care level work. Trainees would be expected to perform personal care tasks alongside qualified and in-service trained staff and to assist in teaching residents through a structured programme of social and personal development. In general the work of Trainees should be selected according to training needs and each trainee should be supported at all times by his study supervisor.

Qualified Staff

287. *Beyond the broad division between Basic Care Staff and qualified staff we saw the need for further divisions among qualified staff.* We envisage the bulk of the work in a mental handicap residential unit being performed by qualified residential care staff. On successful completion of his training the Trainee would move on to the Qualified Care Worker grade at which level he

would perform both basic residential care tasks and developmental tasks with skill and intelligence. After suitable experience and, perhaps, post-qualifying training some Qualified Care Staff might be given additional responsibilities within the unit, or be designated deputy to the Head of a Unit, or become Head of a Unit. Another possibility is that, having undertaken additional training in a particular area of specialisation a Qualified Care Worker might be made responsible for a group of residents with particular problems. In all these cases the Qualified Care Worker should be rewarded financially for the extra duties. *We envisage the Qualified Care Worker grade being used very flexibly to encompass a wide variety of staffing situations from the newly qualified worker to the experienced Unit Head. We do however recognise the need for an additional higher qualified grade at Unit level: we call this the Advanced (Unit) level Care Worker.*

Unit Heads

288. *Each living Unit should have a Unit Head at Qualified Care Worker or Advanced (Unit) Care Worker level.* Unit Heads should spend approximately 40% of their time in direct care of the residents; the rest would be spent on duties which would take them away from direct contact with the residents. Unit Heads would manage and supervise the work of Qualified and Basic Care Staff and Trainees; this would include responsibility for staff development and counselling. They would manage the work of domestic staff (cooks, cleaners etc) employed on the Unit and would be responsible for recruiting them. Unit Heads would co-ordinate advice from other disciplines, and call in outside experts when necessary; organise and play a major role in case conferences; plan and review care programmes and monitor their application. They would be involved in the selection and appointment of Qualified and Basic Care Staff and could bar the appointment of anyone they considered unsuitable. Other duties would include; contributing to the formulation of operational plans and to decision-making on the running of the Unit (within the policies laid down by the employing authority); playing the major, and usually decisive role in decisions on admissions – including short-term "family support" admissions – and transfers of residents, within an agreed but flexible policy; and controlling the domestic arrangements for the Unit. Where common services exist and could not be abolished (or where it would be uneconomic to abandon them) Unit Heads should be able to influence their operation. This might involve co-ordinating the work of domestic and catering staff to fit in with local arrangements; influencing the direction and nature of work done to the buildings and to the grounds by the authority's building contractors and gardeners; and ensuring that each resident has freedom of choice in clothing and personal effects.

289. The decision as to whether a particular unit requires a Qualified Care Worker or Advanced (Unit) Care Worker as Head will depend on such factors as the number of residents in the Unit; the function of the Unit; the degree of responsibility required of the Unit Head; the special needs of the residents; the availability of senior staff support; whether the Unit provides skilled advice and assistance to parents, families and other Units; and the degree of interaction with external professionals. We therefore *RECOMMEND* **that** individual authorities should be left to decide on the appropriate grading for the Head of each individual Unit, with the proviso that **all Unit Heads should be**

qualified mental handicap residential care staff with experience in a residential unit at a lower level. Heads of children's Units, like other qualified staff working in these Units, must have taken the children's module in their training.

Management Grades

290.   *Beyond the Head of Unit we envisage posts in management for qualified and experienced staff. These posts would be at two levels, one contained within the mental handicap field but with responsibility for the provision of advice and management to several Units, and one with responsibilities wider than mental handicap residential care. The first of these we call Advanced (Management) Care Worker and the second Senior Manager.*

291.   We considered whether Advanced (Management) Care Staff should be purely advisers with no management responsibility; staff such as these exist in some local authorities today (although they are usually responsible for a wider field than simply mental handicap residential care) but there is considerable debate about their exact role. A major factor in our decision was the organisational problem arising from the employment of both a non-executive adviser and a line manager responsible for the same service. It is often difficult to clarify where responsibility for decision-making really lies, particularly in defining the adviser's sphere of influence and in establishing the status of his advice. Advisers are inevitably drawn into problems of management and this results not only in conflict between advisers and managers but also in problems in defining areas of responsibility. **We therefore** *RECOMMEND* **that Advanced (Management) Care Staff should have dual responsibility for both management and the quality of service:** decisions affecting the balance between administrative considerations and the quality of care would thus be in the hands of one person.

292.   The duties of Advanced (Management) Care Staff would include: the selection and appointment of Heads of Units; monitoring their performance; systems planning; helping Unit staff to develop operational procedures; advice on programmes for residents; discipline; operation of admissions and discharge procedures within agreed policies; matching staff establishments to needs; and ensuring that relief staff are available in an emergency.

293.   *Senior Managers and above will have responsibilities wider than mental handicap residential care and will need to fit into an existing organisational structure.* In local authorities at present this could mean that a Senior Manager would have responsibility for both day and residential care for mentally handicapped people or alternatively responsibility for the whole field of residential care with all client groups. Similar arrangements are common in the very senior nursing posts in the NHS. We anticipate that in future Senior Managers and above will be responsible for contributing to the comprehensive range of services for mentally handicapped people whether they be general or client group based. Other duties would include involvement in manpower and financial planning across the board, including participation in decision-making about budgets; contribution to forward planning arrangements; membership of joint care planning teams; provision of advice on design planning and architectural briefing in consultation with staff working in direct residential care (ie at Unit level). In the mental handicap field they would be concerned with the inter-relationship between residential care, special education, day

111

care and housing; the level of input of ATC and further education programmes to residential care; the assessment and evaluation of staff; and the monitoring of staff training. Because the responsibilities of Senior Managers may be wider than residential care or mental handicap, holders of these posts will come from a variety of backgrounds, training and experience but we hope and expect that many staff trained and experienced in mental handicap residential care will advance to these higher posts.

Direct Care Staff

294. Our structure is based on the principle of teamwork with staff at all levels working together without demarcation problems. Our model calls for residential care staff to spend the majority of their time and energy in working with the residents. All residents, but particularly children, need to form lasting personal relationships with staff, and we require staff with experience and skill to work in direct residential care. The more work levels there are in a Unit the more remote from the residents and from direct residential care the skilled and experienced worker becomes. A rigid and hierarchical model rewards staff who do well in the basic residential care role by promoting them away from the arena in which their talents are most required. Meanwhile the vital direct residential care role is left to untrained and newly recruited staff. We believe that out teamwork model and our proposed career structure should help to reverse this unfortunate pattern. On the other hand we recognise that to achieve the well trained workforce which we desire would require learners to be withdrawn from direct residential care at frequent intervals for tuition.

Supervision/Management

295. We make a distinction between the supervision and the management of staff. By supervision we mean the provision of broad help and assistance on the job, plus monitoring and assessment of performance. Management implies stricter accountability and should include supervision plus acceptance of responsibility for the work of others, including staff counselling and career development.

Balance Between Staff Levels

296. Having decided on the various staff levels required in mental handicap residential care we then had to decide on appropriate ratios between the various levels. **Given the increased training and the important role we envisage for the new version of the current Nursing and Care Assistant grades we** *RECOMMEND* **a ratio of approximately 1:1 for Basic Care Staff to qualified staff (up to and including Senior Manager). Within Units we envisage a ratio of 1 Qualified Care Worker to 1.3 Basic Care Staff and 1 Advanced (Unit) Care Worker to 2.6 Qualified Care Staff. Thus we** *RECOMMEND* **that 50% of the workforce be qualified and 50% in-service trained.** We believe that this provides reasonable promotion prospects for Qualified Care Staff and ensures adequate supervision. It is difficult to estimate the proportion of Advanced (Management) Care Staff which will be required, since so much will depend on local conditions, *but we envisage at least 2 posts at this level to every 15 Advanced (Unit) Care Staff.*

AN EXAMPLE OF LOCAL SERVICE

297. In the preceding paragraphs we have described the different levels of work required in each Unit and the different levels of skill and training required for staff at each level. We have estimated that a balance of 50% qualified and 50% in-service trained staff will be required, a significant increase on the current numbers of qualified staff. To illustrate how our structure might work in practice we have devised a scheme (Figure 20) for the mental handicap services for a population of 100,000 people. We have estimated the number of mentally handicapped people needing residential services in accordance with White Paper targets although, as we have explained elsewhere, we recognise that these targets are due for review and have quite clearly overestimated the need for children's hospital places. The staff/resident ratio we have used is 1:1 for children and 1:1.5 for adults (see paragraph 181 of Chapter 4), which includes an allowance for night cover. The size of the homes

FIGURE 20 – EXAMPLE OF STAFFING FOR A LOCAL SERVICE

Examples of Residential Units	Places	RESIDENTIAL CARE STAFF NUMBERS (whole time equivalents) Covering 24 hours		
		Basic Care Staff	Qualified Care Staff	Advanced (Unit) Care Staff
ADULTS				
Unit A	24	8	6	2
„ B	24	8	6	2
„ C	12	2	2	1
„ D	12	6	4	1
„ E	12	4	3 ⎫	2
„ F	12	4	3 ⎬	
„ G	8	3	2 ⎫	
„ H	8	3	2 ⎬	2
„ I	8	2	2 ⎭	
CHILDREN				
Unit J	12	6	5	1
„ K	8	4	3	1
„ L	4	2	1	1
Additional Senior Night staff supervising all Units				2
TOTALS	144	52	39	15

The balance between the various levels in this model is:

	Number	%
Advanced (Unit) Care Staff	15	14
Qualified Care Staff	39	37
Basic Care Staff	52	49

113

and the grades of staff suggested to man them in Figure 20 were selected arbitrarily, for illustrative purposes only. They should not be taken to imply endorsement by the Committee of any particular size of Unit or method of staffing. The manpower effort required to satisfy the needs of residents will differ according to local circumstances; what we are suggesting is that overall, in a population Unit of a given size, we see a need for a certain number of staff to serve a prescribed clientele. How these staff are allocated between different Units is for each employing authority to determine.

Representation at Top Levels of Management

298.   We have considered in some detail the various levels of staff which we believe are required to provide a good residential service for mentally handicapped people. At the higher levels we have accepted that responsibilities of staff will encompass either day and residential services for mentally handicapped people or residential services for a variety of client groups including mentally handicapped people. This is similar to the existing structure in local authority services and not dissimilar to the structure starting at Divisional Nursing Officer in the NHS where senior nursing staff often cover services for more than one client group.

299.   In the new mental handicap residential care structure which we are recommending, posts up to and including Advanced (Management) Care Worker will be available in both the NHS and the local authorities. But if mental handicap residential care is to be integrated with the mainstream of residential care the senior posts will, in future, lie in the local authorities. We therefore hope to see a much higher degree of collaboration between health and local authorities not only in the interchange of staff but also in the planning and financing of mental handicap services. Posts at Senior Manager level and beyond will need to be filled by staff with experience in mental handicap services provided by both types of authority. It will be advantageous for staff employed by either health or social services authorities to plan their careers at an early stage to obtain the right mix of qualifications and experience to enable them to progress to the top posts. We believe that the new training and career structure which we are recommending will create wider promotion opportunities for staff at all levels. The implementation of our report will not only provide staff with the prospect of individual responsibility and rewarding and responsible work with mentally handicapped people but will also open up the opportunity of moving into other branches of residential care after a short additional training. We recognise however, that some mental handicap nurses may wish to remain in nursing: we describe the choice for these staff in paragraph 339.

300.   We recognise that our recommendations would create problems in the representation of residential care staff and, indeed, of mental handicap itself, at the higher levels of NHS management particularly at District Management Team and Area and Regional Team of Officers levels. Ideally mental handicap residential care staff would represent themselves at the various management levels just as they would expect to contribute to joint care planning. But because of the relatively small number of staff involved, compared with other staff groups, we recognise that if mental handicap residential care staff were to be given special representation at senior levels other staff groups would quite legitimately ask for a place as well and the whole concept

114

of small planning teams would be lost. Mental handicap has to be represented in some way and we therefore considered whether any of the disciplines now included on planning teams would be able to put the mental handicap point of view. We decided that no one person could do this satisfactorily and that what was required was a reversion to the original idea of these management teams as bearing collective responsibility rather than acting as delegates for particular staff groups. *We do, however, believe that senior mental handicap care staff should be represented on the management teams whenever decisions about mental handicap care are being considered.*

The Area Mental Handicap Services Officer

301. **To achieve this representation we** *RECOMMEND* **the appointment of an Area Mental Handicap Services Officer (AMHSO) who would be accountable directly to the Area Health Authority.** Although not a member of the Area Team of Officers he would receive all the Team papers, and attend meetings as of right whenever a subject to be discussed concerned, or had implications for, mental handicap. He would also have the right to propose matters concerning mental handicap for Team discussion and have the same right of access to the AHA as other members of the Team and other chief professional officers. The grading of this post would vary, at least initially, according to the extent of the mental handicap services. Sometimes it might be at Advanced (Management) level or Senior Manager level, sometimes an Advanced (Unit) level appointment might be more appropriate. In the larger services a District Mental Handicap Services Officer might be appointed with a similar relationship to the District Management Team. In all cases the officer concerned would be nominated by the Authority to perform this representational role in addition to his other duties. The AMHSO would not have any staff management responsibilities, other than those of his primary post as a residential care worker, but would advise the Area Team of Officers on mental handicap residential services. When mental handicap was to be discussed at Regional level one of the Area Mental Handicap Services Officers could be nominated to act additionally at this level.

302. Our recommendation for a new type of mental handicap residential care worker does not have such a major effect on local authority management structures and on the surface these would remain unchanged. But our concern about the representation of mental handicap and of residential care staff at the top management levels applies equally to local authorities. We expect the views and expertise of service providers to be taken into account when new services are planned and planning teams should co-opt staff who have special experience and knowledge. *The person in charge of mental handicap services within a local authority should be of a sufficiently senior level (eg an Assistant Director) for his views to carry weight in the allocation of resources.*

303. Although we have indicated how we see the voice of mental handicap being heard by both health and local authority senior management we do not expect the planning of complementary services to be carried out in isolation; it is important for mental handicap services to be seen as a whole. Joint Care Planning Teams and joint financing are steps in this direction but there is no reason why the Director of Social Services should not attend a meeting of the Area Team of Officers of the AHA, or the Area Mental Handicap Services

Officer of the AHA attend a meeting of the Social Services Committee. We hope that staff will consider the wider field of mental handicap and not just their small part of it.

STAFF MANAGEMENT

Accountability

304.   We do not see it as our job to prescribe in detail the responsibility and accountability of each member of staff – that is the task of local management – but we do believe that it is vitally important for all staff to be very clear about what is expected of them, to whom they are accountable for their actions, and where they can turn when they need help. In our view there are two main ways in which this can be ensured. *First, senior officers should be familiar with the authority's operational policy and should establish for each Unit a clear and unambiguous operational policy, drawn up in collaboration with Unit Heads and Advanced (Management) Care Staff.* This would set out the aims of the Unit and the responsibilities of the Unit Head and his staff as well as detailing what should be expected of the authority itself. Second, *each member of staff should be given a full job description* and this should be considered an essential part of every contract of service.

Individual Responsibility

305.   There are important differences in the way present day residential care staff work and how we see them operating in the future. This is particularly true in the responsibility given to many nurses in large hospitals; the OPCS study shows that large numbers of qualified staff never attend case conferences (OPCS Table 51) and less than half of ward sisters claim to take part in major decisions affecting their patients (such as – whether a new patient should be admitted to or transferred out of their ward, whether a patient should attend a training centre or occupational therapy unit, or whether he should attend school or be allowed to go home at weekends – OPCS Table 53). We expect the residential care worker of the future to have much more individual responsibility, particularly at Head of Unit level; the Unit Head will operate more like the heads of some present day small "hospital hostels" than like the current Charge Nurses of wards in big hospitals. We recognise that some existing staff who have not previously been given the opportunity to participate in decisions about care practices may find this difficult at first but we believe that they will quickly learn the necessary skills and will find their new role more rewarding.

306.   Our model is based on the belief that residents should have as full and rich a life as possible and this demands a good deal from residential care staff. It means far more than ensuring that the clients' physical needs are met: educational, social and recreational needs are equally important. Parents and families have to be encouraged to visit the Units and invited to take part in planning programmes of care for their relatives; and residents have to be encouraged to participate in the life of the community both inside and outside the Unit. In addition, we expect Unit Heads to carry out normal staff management and training responsibilities. One of their important functions in their role as staff managers will be to create the right atmosphere within the Unit.

Effective team work is essential in all Units whatever their size and this will be achieved only if staff work in harmony with each other.

Support

307.   Some care staff are already undertaking many of the tasks which we recommend; where our proposed system differs from the majority of those operating to-day is in giving residential care staff the opportunity of deciding for themselves where and how these tasks can be done without having to refer to others except to ask for professional advice. Thus, although we believe that there will be greater rewards for staff in our model of care we recognise that there will also be a greater burden on individual staff. Residential care staff at all levels must therefore be quite clear as to the extent of their own responsibilities and the responsibilities of others so that they know when it is time to seek further advice. In all areas of work there will be occasions when problems require the consideration of staff with greater experience or authority. At such times it is essential that all staff know where they can turn. For staff below Unit Head, the Head would be the natural source of help but he himself will sometimes need help and there should be a clear and unequivocal point of contact outside the Unit with whom difficult problems can be discussed. This will normally be the Advanced (Management) Care Worker. This person will have similar responsibility for a number of Units and will be able to deal with the problem himself or know how to mobilise additional help.

Risk Taking

308.   Residential care staff will have to implement multi-disciplinary decisions about how far mentally handicapped people can be allowed to act independently, with all that that implies in terms of risk. We have already indicated that we do not want mentally handicapped people to be completely insulated from the day-to-day risks to which everybody else is exposed, but the balance between acceptable risk taking and irresponsibility on the part of residential care staff is a delicate one which varies from case to case. Guidance about risk taking should be included in the Unit's operational policy but the Unit Head will have to take individual decisions after consultation with his own staff, other professional advisers and parents and relatives.

RELATIONSHIPS WITH OTHER PROFESSIONS

309.   In our model of care we have said that mentally handicapped people should have access to public services in the normal way. For those living in residential units this means that the residential care staff must act *in loco parentis* when dealing with these services. The services involved will range from those provided by the Primary Health Care Team, who, together with the psychiatrist, will provide an intermittent service as the occasion demands, to the on-going services such as those provided by social workers or the remedial professions. In many cases what we are recommending is merely a continuation or an extension of the links which have already been built up between residential care staff and staff of other professions, but we are also making some recommendations for changes in interdisciplinary relationships. *The Head of the residential Unit will be the key figure in the new type of service our model of care demands.* Assisted and advised by his staff he will be the

prime mover in organising the services which he believes his residents require. In his dealings with the providers of these services he will be regarded as an equal, as opposed to the subordinate position which he sometimes occupies to-day.

310.   Many residents in mental handicap Units will require the services of the psychiatrist only on an out-patient basis. The psychiatrist has historically played a major decision-making role in the mental handicap hospital and in many cases the organisation of the hospital is such that he is still expected to take the ultimate management responsibility. The role of the psychiatrist is changing, but the hospital management system will have to change too if he is to be freed to undertake wider responsibilities. In the future the psychiatrist will be spending more of his time in work in the community with families, at special schools and ATCs, and in support of other specialist staff. We applaud this change and believe it will not only lead to an improved service for mentally handicapped people outside residential institutions but will also be another step towards normal services for the residents themselves.

311.   The increased contribution of psychology to the care and development of mentally handicapped people has been recognised in a series of recent Government reports[31] [43] [44]. Our model of care requires residential staff who can plan and implement teaching programmes, who can work effectively as members of a team and who can adapt themselves to change. We believe that psychologists have much to offer in advising and supporting these staff in their understanding of themselves, the small groups in which they work and the development of teaching programmes.

312.   The number of social workers attached to mental handicap hospitals is relatively small and we hope that in future it will be possible to link each residential Unit with the Area Social Work Team. It is for the Head of each Unit to request a social work service for his residents not only to provide long term support for the residents and their families but also so that immediate social work intervention is available in emergencies.

313.   The Unit Head must ensure that residents are assessed for their ability to benefit from physiotherapy services and that those who need it receive proper treatment. To ensure maximum and continuing benefit to the residents the physiotherapist should co-operate with the Unit staff to help them understand simple routine procedures which can reinforce the treatment for individual residents. Similar arrangements should be made with the speech and occupational therapists.

314.   Unit Heads should also have regular contacts with the staff of the local special schools, ATCs, and colleges of futher education which some residents will be attending. On occasions liaison will be required with the Disablement Resettlement Officer and the Youth Employment Officer at the local employment services agency, or with the local sheltered workshop. Health care would normally be provided by the local GP who would be contacted by the Unit Head as required. The GP would also provide access to the Health Visitor and Community Nursing Services.

Inter-Disciplinary Work

315.   Although we have described some of the sources of expert advice

118

that Heads of Units may need to call on for their residents that advice cannot be taken in isolation. Advice from one source may lead to the need for help from another source and it is important that staff in residential Units look at each resident in relation to all the services that are available to him. This is probably best done at the time of initial assessment or review when the advice of a variety of experts will be available or on call. The normal procedure for initial assessment and subsequent review will be for inter-disciplinary teams to be convened at regular predetermined intervals, but sometimes additional meetings will be required. Regular meetings have the advantage of a flexible agenda which can be regulated to take account of cases brought forward by individual group members. Meetings for specific purposes can be planned more precisely ensuring that the relevant professional advice is available at the right time with specific expertise co-opted as required. A mixture of both methods is probably necessary but in all cases it will be the Unit Head who will arrange for the meetings to take place and ensure that the right mix of experts is present. The Unit Head and/or members of his staff will be permanent members of these teams.

316.   In addition to this inter-professional co-operation on the part of service providers, mental handicap services also need co-ordinated planning. Residential care should be one element of a unified pattern of services, but too often in the past mentally handicapped people and their families have had to deal with a bewildering variety of agencies. Joint Care Planning Teams and joint financing are beginning to show the way in which the health and personal social services can be co-ordinated across administrative boundaries. The concept of a truly inter-disciplinary service at all levels is not new, but we wish to see it more fully exploited. *There should be regular and frequent contacts between specialist senior staff not only of the health and personal social services but also of housing and education authorities*

Volunteers and Voluntary Organisations

317.   It is important to maintain the distinction between volunteers and voluntary organisations, but both have a vital contribution to make to the welfare of mentally handicapped people. Volunteers, whether as individuals or members of a "League of Friends" or an organisation such as "One-to-One" cannot in any way replace the professional care worker. The volunteer represents the general concern of the community at large, and working in close co-operation with the professionals he can offer friendship and support to residents and their families. Volunteers have made valuable contributions by, for example, befriending hospital patients who would otherwise have had no visitors, organising clubs for mentally handicapped adolescents, and helping residents in homes to integrate into the local community. We wish to encourage all these activities.

318.   Voluntary organisations are of two main types. The first type consists of members with a personal interest in and knowledge of a particular subject, eg organisations of parents of handicapped children. The second type of

voluntary body is geared to providing a service eg Dr Barnado's, (although the first type of voluntary body may also provide a service and employ professionally trained staff). Organisations of the Dr Barnado's type have traditionally provided services of a very high quality, often pioneering new forms of care. Their flexibility and independence have enabled them to experiment and to carry forward thinking in both service and training terms.

319.   There should be a two-way traffic between the Unit on one hand and the volunteers and voluntary organisations on the other, so that outsiders come into the Unit and residents go out into the community. *We look to the Unit Head to ensure that residential care staff and volunteers/staff of voluntary bodies work together to their mutual benefit.*

Parents

320.   As a Committee, we have emphasised the importance of maintaining links between residents and their families and friends. Relatives can not only assist residential care workers to identify the best ways in which residents may be helped but must whenever possible be brought in when any new care programme is being discussed. Residential care staff in their turn will advise on how current programmes in the Unit can be maintained when residents go home for holidays and weekends. Staff must set aside sufficient time for discussions of this kind. Parents, relatives and voluntary bodies can be a powerful force for change and residential care staff should not underestimate their value as lobbyists. *Parents and Unit staff should wherever possible share the task of caring, with unrestricted access by parents and visits from friends and relatives actively encouraged.* In one home we visited the staff told us that the mother of one of the residents came every evening to put her child to bed; this is the sort of shared care we wish to see practised more widely.

STAFF DISCIPLINE

321.   Disciplinary problems can be of 2 kinds: those which relate direct to the job, such as bad timekeeping; and those which relate to professional standards, such as bad practice or conduct unbecoming to the profession. The first problem is a matter of staff management; the second problem, although it too involves management, is more complex.

322.   The GNCs at present have disciplinary powers over the professional standards of mental handicap nurses; there is no comparable watchdog for residential care staff employed by local authorities. Both groups of staff are of course covered by employment protection legislation. A nurse who had been removed from the GNC Register or Roll would no longer be able to practise as a nurse (he might however quite legitimately take on a job in a local authority home since he would not then be being employed as a nurse). Local authorities rely on qualifications and the use of references to maintain standards. We considered in detail the problem of disciplinary powers in relation to professions and concluded that *such vulnerable residents as mentally handicapped people need some form of protection.* Means must be found to ensure that clients receive a minimum standard of service from adequately trained staff and that all clients are protected (in so far as any disciplinary procedure

can offer protection) from staff misconduct in the professional context. **We strongly** *RECOMMEND* **that the employers and professional associations concerned should consider the problem of disciplinary powers and agree on a system of professional discipline at the earliest possible opportunity.**

ASSIMILATING THE EXISTING STAFF

323. In order to achieve the new structure which we have proposed the existing staff must be assimilated to the new grades. In the proposals on assimilation which follow we have been primarily concerned with levels of work; it is not for us to make recommendations about salary structures and conditions of service. Nevertheless we have had to take account of the differences in salaries which exist at present both within and between the health and personal social services, for mental handicap residential care staff. We believe that it should be possible to implement our recommendations without creating anomalies in terms of salaries or grading. The freedom of movement between the NHS and the personal social services which is necessary for the career structure we propose would be very difficult to achieve if the salaries and conditions of service in the two sectors differed. We recognise that these matters are outside our remit and can be agreed only by the relevant negotiating bodies. **We nonetheless strongly** *RECOMMEND* **that these bodies should work towards a unified salary structure and common conditions of service for mental handicap residential care staff in the NHS and in social services departments at the earliest possible opportunity.** The career structure which we have proposed is dependent on residential care workers being able to move easily between living Units run by the NHS (eg in large hospitals) and by social services departments. The perpetuation of separate salaries and conditions would encourage staff to stay within one of the two sectors thus making it difficult for health service staff to transfer to the local authorities at the Advanced (Management) care worker grade.

Basic Care Staff

324. Our proposed Basic Care Worker grade would equate with the present Nursing Assistant and Unqualified Care Assistant grades. *Assimilation at this level could thus be accomplished fairly easily by renaming existing Nursing Assistants and Unqualified Care Assistants as Basic Care Staff.* These staff will in future receive a significant in-service training to equip them to be members of the caring team. *The Basic Care Worker is an important member of that team and his salary and conditions of service should reflect his status in the residential care structure.*

Qualified and Unqualified Staff

325. Our proposed structure calls for an all qualified profession, excluding Basic Care Staff, but many of the current posts which approximate to our Qualified and Advanced (Unit) Care Worker grades are held by staff with no qualification, or an inappropriate qualification. Clearly for some years there will be a shortage of appropriately qualified staff. In considering how existing workers can be assimilated into the new structure we have accepted that there must be an interim phase during which unqualified staff will be recruited to

grades which would eventually be restricted to qualified staff. The length of this interim period will depend upon the speed at which the new training is introduced but **we** RECOMMEND **that each employing authority should set a date after which it will not recruit unqualified or unsuitably qualified staff to the Qualified Care Worker grade and above.** The terms and conditions of service of existing staff must however be protected; *at the end of the interim period all staff in Qualified Care Worker posts and above would be accepted as 'qualified staff'. During and after the interim period these existing staff would be awarded the pay, terms and conditions of service and prospects appropriate to qualified staff.*

326.   Our survey shows (OPCS Tables 15 and 16) that a variety of qualifications are held by nursing and home staff working in the residential care of mentally handicapped people. In nursing the relevant qualifications for mental handicap care are clearly RNMS/RNMD and SEN(MS)/Enrolled Nurse, but in the personal social services the picture is not so clear. The CQSW has been primarily a field social work qualification (although in recent years many CQSW courses have put considerable effort into the development of teaching and practice placements appropriate to the needs of residential workers) and it does not provide specialist teaching on specific client groups (such as elderly or mentally handicapped people). The CRSW, CRCCYP and SCRCCYP are all residential care qualifications but are due to be replaced in 1978 or 1980 by the CSS or CQSW; the CRSW is a generic training but the other two focus on the residential care of children and young people. While it is clearly up to each employing authority to decide which qualifications it will recognise as "appropriate" once the interim period is over **we** RECOMMEND **that recognition should be limited to the following:**

> **CSS (our proposed mental handicap residential care version only)**
>
> **RNMS (RNMD in Scotland)**
>
> **SEN(MS) (Enrolled Nurse in Scotland)**
>
> **CQSW (only if sufficient specialist work has been undertaken –** *see Chapter 5, paragraph 245)*
>
> **Specific CSS/CQSW courses which replaced CRSW, CRCCYP or SCRCCYP courses.**

Qualified Care Staff

327.   In nursing at present there are three types of staff at roughly Qualified Care Worker level: Enrolled Nurses, Senior Enrolled Nurses and Staff Nurses (RNMS/RNMD). In salary terms Staff Nurse/Senior Enrolled Nurse is similar to qualified or unqualified Group Leader/Assistant Officer-in-Charge in the local authorities. We considered two alternatives for the assimilation of existing staff to the Qualified Care Worker grade. One possibility would be to designate Enrolled Nurses, Staff Nurses, Senior Enrolled Nurses and Group Leaders/Assistant Officer-in-Charge (qualified and unqualified) as Qualified Care Staff. Local authority unqualified staff and Enrolled Nurses would be debarred from progressing beyond a certain point on the salary scale, while Senior Enrolled Nurses, Staff Nurses and local authority qualified Assistant Officers-in-Charge would be able to continue to the top of the scale without a bar. The other solution would be to assimilate: Enrolled Nurses, Senior

Enrolled Nurses, Staff Nurses and qualified or unqualified Group Leaders and Assistant Officers-in-Charge, to the Qualified Care Worker grade and, after an interim period, to limit recruitment or promotion to any qualified grade to those with a recognised qualification (see paras 325 and 326). **We prefer to** *RECOMMEND* **the second possibility because we do not wish to see a distinction in status between different staff doing the same job.**

Deputies

328. The post of Deputy Officer-in-Charge in local authority homes is roughly equivalent to that of Deputy Charge Nurse (a grade which is not in common use) in the health service. *Our structure does not provide specifically for Deputy Unit Heads although we have suggested that one of the Qualified Care Staff could be nominated Deputy and given an allowance.* This should not present any assimilation problems.

Advanced (Unit) Care Staff

329. We envisage the Advanced (Unit) Care Worker as the Head of a small living Unit. In the local authorities this would equate to the Head of Home while the NHS equivalent would be Ward Sister/Charge Nurse. In salary terms however the Officer-in-Charge equates more nearly to Nursing Officer I and II. It would be possible to create a long salary scale to accommodate all these grades and to divide this long scale into smaller bands according to the size and type of living Unit as is the practice in the local authorities. In this way the more junior staff (Sisters and Charge Nurses) could be paid the lower salary appropriate to Heads of smaller living Units while the more senior staff (Nursing Officers) could be assimilated onto the top end of the scale as Heads of larger living Units. This would however encourage Advanced (Unit) Care Staff to move up the ladder from small Units to large Units in order to increase their salaries. Apart from being damaging to continuity of care this would create the erroneous impression that small Units were less of a challenge to run than large Units. *We would prefer to see the employing authorities and staff unions coming together to agree on some financial means of rewarding experienced workers without the need to move from Unit to Unit.* Similarly promotion away from direct care (ie to Advanced (Management) Care Worker) should not be the only means of financial advancement for Advanced (Unit) Care Staff and **we would therefore prefer to see overlapping pay scales for these two grades. Another method of rewarding experienced residential care workers would be the use of accelerated increments. We** *RECOMMEND* **that the Advanced (Unit) Care Worker grade should comprise:**

> **Ward Sisters/Charge Nurses**
> **Some Nursing Officers**
> **Officers-in-Charge**

The present Nursing Officer grade would be assimilated to the Advanced (Unit) or Advanced (Management) grades depending on current practice, ie Nursing Officers in charge of large "Salmon Units" (120–140 beds) would become Advanced (Management) Care Staff and those in charge of smaller Salmon Units would become Advanced (Unit) Care Staff.

123

Unit Heads

330. All staff involved in providing a service to mentally handicapped people will have to re-assess their roles within the new system of care which we are proposing, but those nurses who will become Unit Heads are likely to be the most affected by the changes. *Our recommendations require substantial delegation of powers and duties from existing Senior Nursing Officers and Nursing Officers to Ward Sisters/Charge Nurses.* This delegation could not be accomplished overnight and will need to be carefully planned. Initially it may prove easier to delegate responsibility for Unit policy than to give Unit Heads control over practical matters such as duty rosters and staff appointments. In the early stages the Unit Head might take over the co-ordination of treatment and care programmes for the residents, become the convenor of multi-disciplinary meetings, and play a major role in making decisions on admissions and discharges. Senior management will need to ensure that this new, more active role for existing Ward Sisters/Charge Nurses is fully understood by other members of the team.

Advanced (Management) Care Staff

331. In our structure the Advanced (Management) Care Worker would be an adviser and manager responsible for a number of small mental handicap living Units. Some local authorities have a Homes Adviser but this post is not strictly comparable to our Advanced (Management) Care Worker. **For assimilation purposes however, existing Homes Advisers, some Nursing Officers and some Senior Nursing Officers could be transferred to the Advanced (Management) Care Worker grade. We** *RECOMMEND* **that there should be an overlap in the salary scales for the Advanced (Management) grade and the Senior Manager grade and that SNOs should be assimilated to either level according to current practice.**

Senior Managers

332. The Senior Manager would be responsible either for domiciliary, day, and residential services for mentally handicapped people or (in local authorities only), for residential services for all client groups. The post would be roughly equivalent to Divisional Nursing Officer in the NHS and Principal Officer (Residential and Day Services) in the local authorities. **We** *RECOMMEND* **that staff in both these existing grades be assimilated as Senior Managers.**

A NATIONAL STAFF COMMISSION

333. The introduction of the structure we propose would present difficult practical problems and health and social service authorities would need guidance on the detailed implementation of our proposals. **We** *RECOMMEND* **that a National Staff Commission be established to supervise the introduction of our proposals and to adjudicate on any complaints from existing staff. We strongly** *RECOMMEND* **that existing staff be treated generously in the implementation of our structure.** No member of staff need fear that his pay and conditions will be worsened by our proposals.

Size

334.   In Chapter 3, in describing our concept of small group living, we said that large institutions – including homes of 20 or more beds – would be with us for many more years. But the concept of a small, intimate living group can and indeed must be created within existing, seemingly unfavourable, surroundings. *Some hospital wards are already operating as semi-autonomous Units and we depend upon further progress in this direction.* Smallness should not be regarded as an end in itself, but a ward or living group which functions independently can help to prevent the staff and residents from becoming institutionalised. Imaginative use of existing facilities and well thought out upgrading schemes can encourage the scale reduction which our model requires. The National Development Group's hospital study[21] has some excellent practical advice on "creating a home" in hospital, and Maureen Oswin[29] has shown some of the consequences of failing to do so. Both these studies are as relevant to local authority homes as to hospitals.

335.   The needs of the residents and local constraints will clearly have a major effect in determining the exact size of living groups. A group home would probably be smaller than a Unit for profoundly handicapped adults and an autonomous living group within a large hospital or home would be subject to quite different constraints on size from those governing an independent building. We have been very much encouraged by examples of collaboration between social services departments, housing departments and voluntary housing associations in the provision of group living accommodation. There is potential for a great increase in schemes of this kind which add to the range of ordinary living experiences open to mentally handicapped people and reduce their dependence on the more expensive and isolating specialist homes. Health and social services authorities should be constantly on the look-out for opportunities to provide independent housing, with or without unobtrusive supervision. *No mentally handicapped person who is able to do so should be deprived of the opportunity to look after himself.*

A Real Home

336.   In a real home everyone shares the jobs to be done and the facilities available. Staff attitudes will, in many cases, have to change if hospitals and residential homes are to achieve this atmosphere of sharing. The first priority for residential care staff is to enable the residents to look after themselves, but essential physical care tasks have been turned into routines, with the residents being treated *en bloc*, to the exclusion of true care. Chronic understaffing means, for example, that the nurses on a hospital ward who succeed in getting all the patients up in the morning are unable to interact with them because they (the nurses) have then to make all the beds. Interaction with the residents should not debar the staff from doing physical tasks for them, but activities such as tidying the ward, bed-making and sorting laundry usually exclude the residents. In this as in all aspects of our model the Unit operational policy should allow for the maximum flexibility, with residents participating in the maintenance of their environment but not being exploited, and domestic staff freeing residential care staff of inappropriate duties without the intrusion of an army of cooks, cleaners and bed-makers to disrupt Unit life.

337. Routine physical tasks are both a symptom and a result of the institutional approach to care. Many mental handicap hospital wards still appear to be run according to clinical standards of tidiness, with furniture neatly and symmetrically arranged and few personal possessions (other than wall posters) visible. Older staff in particular may find it hard to accept that professional standards of care can be maintained in a ward which looks "lived in". We are not advocating dirty wards or slovenly care practices but we do condemn the obsessive pursuit of uniformity and barren tidiness (although we recognise that overcrowding and understaffing have made these features a necessity in some cases). The hospital ward or local authority home is "home" to those mentally handicapped children and adults who live there and both staff and residents will find it easier to accept this if the place looks homely.

Uniforms

338. In an ordinary home people do not wear uniforms, but according to our survey (OPCS para 5.6) about 80% of nursing staff and 40% of local authority residential care staff wear them. We are aware of the long running debate on the need for uniforms in mental handicap hospitals; the subject arouses high feelings and a tendency to make dogmatic assertions, but it is by no means a simple problem. Some people argue that uniforms are necessary to maintain social distance between staff and residents, to emphasise the authority of staff and to provide a visual indication of the place of each staff member in the hierarchy. Others argue that social distance, authority and hierarchies are not merely irrelevant to mental handicap residential care but positively damaging to it. The debate is further complicated by the financial aspects of the problem. **We recognise that protective clothing may sometimes be necessary and we** *RECOMMEND* **that direct residential care staff be given a clothing allowance and permitted to choose whether to wear a uniform/overall.** The traditional nursing uniform is, however, quite inappropriate for mental handicap residential care staff.

THE CHOICE FOR NURSES

339. For mental handicap nurses our proposals will mean more than a new approach to the job, they will also mean a new professional identity. We believe that the majority of mental handicap nurses will see our proposals as helping them to give a better service to their residents, and will be willing to take on the new role of residential care worker as part of the package. We recognise, however, that some staff may be unwilling to sever their links with the nursing profession and may prefer instead to move out of mental handicap residential care and into some other branch of nursing. The wishes of these staff should be respected. There are already shortened courses of training for nurses wanting to transfer from one part of the Register or Roll to another. **We** *RECOMMEND* **that any mental handicap nurse who prefers to remain in nursing should be offered every assistance to obtain a place on one of these courses.**

340. In the changeover from mental handicap nurse to mental handicap residential care worker there are many problems of pay and conditions which will have to be resolved. These problems include the Mental Health Officer status and the psychiatric "lead" (additional salary) held by mental handicap nurses, and the status of the mental handicap parts of the Register and Roll.

126

These issues and many others can be resolved only by discussions between all those concerned, including trade unions, employers and professional bodies. Although we are not able to offer any solutions **we strongly** *RECOMMEND* **that the proposed National Staff Commission be asked to consider these issues at the earliest possible opportunity and to ensure that no existing member of staff will lose by our recommendations.**

CHAPTER 7 – FINANCE AND PRIORITIES

INTRODUCTION

341.   We realised from the start that our recommendations would be expensive in terms of both financial and real resources. Mental handicap services have received a high priority in recent years but the exceptional growth rate which has been permitted must be placed in the context of the very low baseline from which the services have had to develop. We believe that we have made the case for increasing mental handicap's share of national resources but we feel it would be irresponsible to make resource-intensive recommendations without attempting to place them within the context of the resources which are likely to be available in future years.

342.   The main additional costs will arise on manpower, because of improved staff/resident ratios, and on training, because the CSS is more expensive than nurse training and because there will be more people to train. But our recommendations have financial implications in a number of other areas: for local education authorities, because of the extra college places and teaching staff; for those authorities which will have to provide additional staff to man the essential back-up services; and for health and social services authorities, because of the proposals for small group living and for restructuring the organisation of care staff. Not all of these costs would be incurred at the same time, some would build up gradually over the years, others would fall to be met before the main recruitment and training efforts could begin. On the other hand there would also be savings: the predicted decline in the birthrate (up to the 1990s), the development of services such as fostering and group homes, and the use of existing houses instead of purpose-built accommodation, would all reduce both capital and revenue expenditure on residential services. Depending on the type and extent of handicap, preventive measures too may show a very favourable economic return, since the costs of handicap including for example the costs of lifetime care, are substantial. (Some detailed studies of the economic aspects of prevention have recently been undertaken by the French government and these studies are usefully summarised by Margaret and Arthur Wynn in "Prevention of Handicap of Perinatal Origin"[45].) It would be difficult if not impossible to cost many of these changes and we have therefore concentrated on the two major quantifiable areas of manpower and training.

MANPOWER AND TRAINING COSTS

343.   We considered a possible timetable for the introduction of our manpower and training proposals. This timetable assumed a rapid increase in recruitment and a rapid expansion in training so that our targets could be reached within 14 years. Using average salary cost figures we calculated (for Great Britain) the annual additional cost of our manpower recommendations against a prediction of what might have happened if our Committee had never been appointed. On this plan (in which year one is the first year of the full implementation of our proposals) the costs would rise rapidly over the 13 year period to reach a peak of £84m in year 13. Over the 13 years the total additional cost would be £682m. Additional training costs would increase the

peak figure by £17–£24m and the total cost by £169–£249m. This timetable would be costly, but it must be seen in perspective: in 1976/7 alone £5,608m was spent on revenue account in the health and personal social services.

344.   The DHSS issues annual planning guidelines (for England) giving projected expenditure by health and social services authorities. The latest guidelines (issued in 1978) give projections up to 1981/2. So that we could compare our manpower and training additional costs with the money which was likely to be available for mental handicap residential services we needed to extend the projections to 1991/2. We therefore assumed that the growth rates forecast for mental handicap services up to 1981/2 would continue at the same level until 1991/2. The result of this assumption is shown in Figure 21 below.

FIGURE 21 – REVENUE EXPENDITURE ON MENTAL HANDICAP (ENGLAND)

	Actual expenditure 1976/7	DHSS Projection of Expenditure 1981/2	Jay Projection of Expenditure 1991/2	DHSS/JAY Projected Increase in Expenditure 1976/7-1991/2	
NHS In-Patient and Out-Patient	£189m	£209m	£255m	£66m	
					£115m
Local Authority Residential Care	£22m	£32m	£71m	£49m	
Local Authority Day care	£30m	£41m	£73m	£43m	
Total	£241m	£282m	£399m	£158m	

Our proposals call for additional expenditure, for Great Britain, on manpower and training alone of almost £1,000m over the 13 years, whilst an extrapolation of the forecast growth rates implies an increase in available funds for all aspects of mental handicap residential care of £115m in England over the period 1976/7 to 1991/2. Thus even allowing for the additional funds available for Scotland and Wales (and England accounts for almost 90 per cent of GB residential provision for mental handicap) the 13 year timetable is clearly quite unachievable without a considerable injection of funds. If such funds could be made available we nonetheless doubt whether the new training programme could be got off the ground or the additional manpower recruited over such a short period. In addition there is the problem of accommodation; extra staff could not be recruited without buildings for them to work in. Our recommendations thus have major implications for capital as well as revenue expenditure. It was clear to us from the figures that a 13 year timetable for implementation was quite unrealistic.

A Realistic Strategy

345.   We now had to find an alternative strategy for implementing our proposals. One of the main reasons why the 13 year plan was unrealistic was that it was based on staffing alone, without reference to the provision of the buildings in which the staff would work. We decided that a more realistic approach would be to work out how quickly the services could be developed and calculate staffing and training improvements from a service base.

129

346. Since we would be forecasting services for many years ahead we decided that the best available indicators were the White Paper targets, however suspect some of these now appear, which would take us up to 1991*. We used 1981 as our base year on the assumption that a Government decision on our proposals could not be expected before late 1979 or early 1980 (after the consultation process).

347. The White Paper targets apply to England and Wales only, while DHSS planning guidelines are limited to England and our remit covers Great Britain (ie England, Wales, and Scotland). We decided to use the White Paper targets for places per 100,000 population, calculate these on the forecast England population for 1991 and use England only for our financial calculations. We thought that this would produce a more accurate picture than if we attempted to gross up existing figures to include Scotland and Wales. We realise however that priorities for expenditure in Scotland and Wales may differ somewhat from the English priorities.

348. On the assumptions given in the previous paragraph we estimated that the number of mental handicap residential places required in England in 1991 would be as in Figure 22 below.

FIGURE 22 – ESTIMATED MENTAL HANDICAP RESIDENTIAL PLACES REQUIRED IN 1991 – ENGLAND

	Children	Adults	Total
Social Services Authorities	5,000	29,000	34,000
Health Authorities	4,000*	26,000	30,000
Total	9,000	55,000	64,000

*Based on actual residents under 16 in 1976 (4,263) which should have reduced still further by 1991. The White Paper target of 6,000 overestimated the demand.

On current practice, of the 34,000 places to be provided by local authorities, only 24,000 would be provided in homes actually run by local authorities, the remaining 10,000 being supplied by voluntary and privately run homes. Throughout our report we have tried not to make a distinction between health and social services provision, but we have had to do so in relation to financial matters. The financing arrangements of the two types of authority are quite different and entirely separate. In addition, the White Paper figures which we are using separate the two types of provision.

NHS Mental Handicap Residential Provision (All figures relate to *England only*)

349. The latest (1975) estimated nursing staff/patient ratio is 1:2.1 and we thought it reasonable to assume that a ratio of 1:1.6 could be reached by 1991. This would require 20,000 care staff in 1991, ie 10,000 qualified staff and 10,000 Basic Care staff. These figures are very similar to the number of nursing staff currently (1976) employed in mental handicap hospitals. Since the number of patients in mental handicap hospitals is declining (see Figure 7) an improvement in the staff/resident ratio to 1:1.6 could be achieved by 1991 without increasing the number of care staff. In practice, recruitment would need to continue until the patient population reached the White Paper

*Throughout this Chapter where we have used the calendar year this relates to the financial year starting in April of that year, ie 1991 = financial year 1991/2.

level.* This would, however, depend on the patient population reducing at the rate envisaged in the White Paper; unfortunately the decline has been slower than anticipated. In addition to the qualified staff and Basic Care staff hospitals would also need to employ Trainees. An annual Trainee intake of about 1,750 would be required to maintain 10,000 qualified staff; this would give an annual total of 3,500 Trainees in post.

350.   From our extrapolation of the DHSS planning guidelines we have calculated that if growth continued at the forecast rate, £255m would be available for hospital revenue expenditure on mental handicap in 1991 (see Figure 21). Currently about 44% of mental handicap hospital revenue expenditure is spent on nursing staff. Even if this percentage remained the same in 1991, rather than increasing as might be expected, there would be £112m available for expenditure on direct care staff. The annual cost (November 1976 prices) of 10,000 qualified staff, 10,000 Basic Care staff and 3,500 Trainees would be about £63m.† Additional training costs, since CSS is more expensive than nurse training, would add another £5–£8m per year, depending on the length of the course. Thus the total manpower and training expenditure of £71m could be offset against estimated available resources of £112m. These calculations are shown in Figure 23 below.

FIGURE 23 – MANPOWER AND TRAINING COSTS IN 1991 (ENGLAND)

Available Funds	£m	Costs	£m
Total residential mental handicap revenue budget	255	Residential care staff manpower costs	63
Residential care staff revenue budget	112	Residential care staff training costs	5–8
Total revenue budget available for residential care staff	112A	Total residential care staff costs ..	68–71B

Difference between A and B = £41–£44m (ie unallocated revenue)

Thus the £41–£44m unallocated revenue could be used to move towards the staff ratios used in the "Sheffield Method" (see Chapter 4)‡, which would cost £83m to implement in full in 1991. Alternatively, Ministers might decide to

---

*In order to calculate staffing costs we have had to use staff/resident ratios. These ratios provide a crude indicator of staffing levels but they are subject to a number of important limitations. Our survey shows (OPCS para 3.4) that there is a considerable difference between ratios of staff in post and ratios of staff on duty. In the health service the nursing staff ratios include "administrative" nurses (ie Nursing Officers and above) and also nurse teaching staff, while the local authority figures cover only care staff up to and including Warden/Officer-in-Charge. In a hospital the nursing staff will be unevenly distributed through the wards, according to the age and degree of handicap of the patients. In local authority homes the majority of the residents leave the unit during the day and a large number of part-time staff help out in the morning and evening peak hours. Hospital patients spend more time on the ward and staff are therefore required throughout the day. For these and other reasons the nurse/patient ratio may appear to be more favourable than it in fact is in practice and it is therefore not possible to compare NHS and local authority staff ratios.

†Staff costs are based on equivalent nurse (average) salaries at November 1976 weighted to take account of our proposed grades and staff numbers, including 15% to cover superannuation and employers' National Insurance Contributions.

‡Our target of 60,000 residential care staff is a national total and we do not recommend particular staffing ratios which could be used locally. But to estimate the cost of our proposals we had to use staffing ratios, and for this purpose we used the "Sheffield Method" ratios of 1:1 for children and 1:1.5 for adults because they provided a simple basis for calculations. Individual authorities will need to decide on their own staffing ratios within the total of staff available nationally.

plan for slower growth in health service revenue and a corresponding increase in allocations to local authorities, which would be used either to improve their staffing ratios or to increase numbers in training. But we recognise that if the numbers in hospital continue to decline at the present (slow) rate there will be less unallocated revenue available for such purposes.

Training of NHS Residential Care Staff

351. With the new residential care staff in hospitals no longer to be trained by the GNCs some other means of financing training for health service staff must be found. One solution would be for health authorities to second staff for training on CSS courses, paying the Trainee's salary and training costs. Clearly, RHAs would need to be allocated sufficient funds to pay for this secondment.

SOCIAL SERVICES PROVISION
(All figures relate to *England* only)

352. Paragraphs 349–351 show that in the health service staffing levels and training could be either maintained or improved within the forecast revenue budget for mental handicap hospital services. Since increased expenditure would be more valuable to the personal social services than to the NHS it would be possible to reduce the proposed growth rates for the NHS and increase those for the social services. Of course, such a proposal would need to be set against general resource constraints and since our figures are merely rough estimates we have not included this possibility in our calculations. In the local authorities mental handicap residential care services start from a much lower level of provision and progress towards the White Paper targets for residential places and our proposed staffing levels will be much more difficult to attain.

Possible Staff/Resident Ratios

353. The White Paper forecast a need for 34,000 residential places in 1991. Progress to date (latest figures, 1976) is roughly on target, with adult places above target and children's places below target. Beyond 1976 we have estimated likely revenue expenditure as for the health service, using the DHSS planning guidelines. On this basis £71m might be available for local authority total revenue expenditure on mental handicap. Adjusting this figure to allow for the 10,000 places which would be paid for by local authorities but provided by voluntary and private organisations reduces this to about £50m of which approximately half (£25m) would be available for expenditure on residential care staff. Using average salary costs for residential care staff, this £25m would finance about 9,000 staff at an average staff/resident ratio of about 1:2.65. The salaries of Trainees and the cost of training are not included in these calculations; if they are included the number of residential care staff we could afford would be reduced and the staff/resident ratio worsened.

354. Although a ratio of 1:2.65 is much lower than the "Sheffield Method" ratios it is nonetheless an improvement on the existing ratio of 1:2.77 (England and Wales). On the other hand, the present local authority home population is predominantly mildly handicapped, so that the high staff ratios looked for in mental handicap hospitals would not necessarily be expected in local au-

thority homes at present, whereas by 1991 we expect to see many more people who are severely handicapped living in local authority homes. By 1991 local authority homes may thus be needing much higher staff ratios than those which they have at present. None of the local authority staff ratios quoted take account of the contributions made by day care staff, whereas the nursing staff ratios will often include nurses performing day care activities.

355.   In addition to the ratio of 1:2.65 which could be achieved within forecast expenditure we have also calculated the costs of alternative staffing ratios, both better (1:2) and worse (1:3), and of the "Sheffield Method" ratios (1:1 for children and 1:1.5 for adults). All four ratios are shown in the graph at Figure 24. It will be for the Government to decide which of these ratios, if any, it wishes to aim for but **we strongly *RECOMMEND* that the "Sheffield Method" ratios be introduced nationally as quickly as possible.**

356.   Although the White Paper targets are national forecasts which may not always apply locally we did attempt to estimate the costs of the various staffing ratios for a local authority with a population of 500,000. The results, which should be treated with caution, are shown on the right hand side of the graph at Figure 24.

Training Costs

357.   Given that the White Paper targets for residential places can be met and the existing staff ratio improved (although not up to the "Sheffield Method" ratios) within projected revenue expenditure the major financial problem for local authorities will be the cost of training. At an estimated cost of £4,650–£6,450 per student our training recommendations would cost £19–£26m at the worst (1:3) staff ratio. These training costs cover only the costs to the employing authority, including the employment of study supervisors and replacement staff, but there will be other costs involved in running the new training. We have assumed (for the purpose of our calculations) that the educational costs of CSS would be £1,500 per student although they are likely to be higher, and there are costs involved in training the course tutors and practice supervisors, and in planning CSS courses. Initial planning costs are estimated at £10,000 for each course (although this figure, too, is likely to be on the low side); some assistance with these costs can, however, be provided by DHSS.

358.   Local authorities have to start not only from a shortage of residential homes but also from a low level of qualified staff (and some of these have inappropriate qualifications) within those homes. In 1976 the Birch report, "Manpower and Training for the Social Services"[38], produced proposals to attempt to remedy the shortage of qualified staff in all types of personal social services provision in the UK. There is still a long way to go before the high hopes of the Birch Working Party are fulfilled and there remains a large backlog of staff requiring training which can only be exacerbated by our proposals. Indeed, as CCETSW informed us, there would be a danger of mental handicap care staff upsetting the balance on some CSS courses.

359.   *We believe that unless there is some fundamental rethinking of the present financial arrangements for training in the personal social services there is no hope of achieving an adequate number of trained staff, let alone the highly*

133

FIGURE 24 – LOCAL AUTHORITY MENTAL HANDICAP RESIDENTIAL CARE SERVICES

(cumulative progress to White Paper targets at uniform percentage annual increase of places)

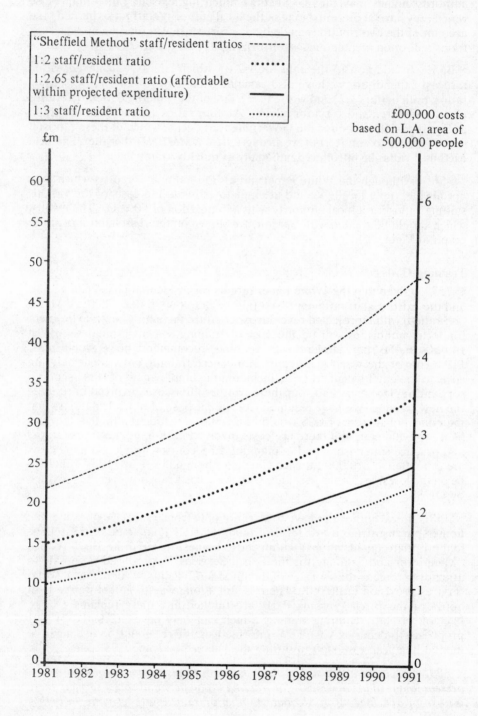

"Sheffield Method" staff/resident ratios   --------
1:2 staff/resident ratio   •••••••
1:2.65 staff/resident ratio (affordable within projected expenditure)   ——————
1:3 staff/resident ratio   ••••••••••

£00,000 costs based on L.A. area of 500,000 people

£m

professional workforce which we see as both necessary and desirable. It is impractical to expect local authorities to increase expenditure on mental handicap staff training at the expense of other staff groups, even given that both central and local government already recognise mental handicap as a high priority after years of neglect. In the personal social services there is no tradition of a fully qualified profession aided by unqualified assistants (as there is in nursing) and no specific mental handicap residential care training. With a shortage of trained staff and of money there will always be temptations to local authorities to recruit unqualified or inappropriately qualified staff rather than spend money on training.

Special Funding

360.   At present, funds for local authority staff training are channelled through the Rate Support Grant system and there is no means of ensuring that the money is actually spent on the purpose intended. If the Government is persuaded to find additional resources to meet our training proposals it would, in our view, be inappropriate for these resources to be fed through the RSG system, in which there would be no certainty that they would be spent on training.

361.   The Birch Working Party met similar difficulties in trying to suggest ways of financing their plans for a greatly increased programme of social services training. They considered a number of possible solutions:–

> a centralised system of Government financial support for all aspects of training; the transfer to central Government of some of the responsibilities at present met by local authorities; the setting up of pooling arrangements for meeting certain training costs; and the introduction of a limited degree of special funding.

For a variety of reasons, particularly lack of enthusiasm from local authority associations at that time, the Working Party made no specific recommendation on any of these possibilities.

362.   But Birch did make one recommendation for financing training. This was that a fund, drawn from both central and local sources, should be established to underwrite certain key aspects of training. *We believe that such a fund is also relevant to our proposed mental handicap training and could meet the cost of, say, training and employing practice supervisors and tutors, and employing replacement staff. Alternatively, the fund could be used to pay for the additional college tutors required for the CSS.* These will be major items in the change to the new form of training and will be difficult if not impossible to meet without some form of central and protected assistance. **We therefore** *RECOMMEND* **that such a fund be established.** There are precedents for special funding in the field of probation and child care training in the 1960s, when changes being implemented were beyond the financial capacity of local services and were made possible by the allocation of central funds. Central funding will also provide a bridge between the two autonomous service employers, health and social services, operating within different financial systems; some form of central assistance will help to remove the present incompatibility between their funding methods. Special funding of this kind can be seen as an interim measure to get the new training system off the ground. We envisage

that after a few years, once the new training has been developed and is seen to be working properly, the special funding could be discontinued and a more locally accountable form of financing training introduced.

The Education Service

363.   Present plans for the education service envisage no increase in total numbers of academic staff in further and higher education up to 1981 and the prospects of increases beyond that time are very uncertain, particularly in view of the forecasts of reduced student numbers and the likely pattern of further and higher education in the 1980s and 1990s. We believe that some of the spare capacity in further education, in terms of both buildings and staff, which is forecast to occur in the late 1980s and early 1990s should be used for mental handicap residential care staff training. But even if the staff can be found there remains the cost of preparation or training for tutors and supervisors on what is to be a specially adapted type of CSS programme. The possibility of a future requirement for compulsory teacher training for new entrants to full-time teaching in further education is an additional problem with cost implications (see para 261).

364.   One way of easing the situation would be to make as much use as possible of the existing nurse education facilities, including the nurse teaching staff, who we hope will continue to work in a different, but equally important role. There seems no reason why mental handicap nurse training schools could not be converted for use as CSS training centres (in place of Colleges of Further Education), using both the equipment and, after reorientation training, many of the staff. Such centres would be run jointly by health, social services and education authorities. Since the GNCs would no longer be organising mental handicap nurse training there might be some very marginal savings from the GNCs' budgets. But CSS training is more expensive than nurse training and the most significant additional expense is the cost of replacement staff, an item which does not arise in the present training of nurses.

OTHER FINANCIAL ASPECTS

365.   We have discussed the problems for local social services authorities of financing our manpower and training recommendations and mentioned the capital costs of providing small units. In the health service too there will be costs involved in setting up the small living units which our model of care requires; there are also cost implications for education. But our recommendations are only part of the total mental handicap service and our claims must be put alongside the claims of the rest of the service. Residential care services and residential care staff training cannot be looked at in isolation from services such as day nurseries, part time residential care, baby sitting services, home helps, special education, day care, and voluntary and parent groups. The development of each of these goes hand in hand with the development of residential services and indeed spending on these may mean that dependence on residential care could be reduced.

366.   There are other implications even beyond the narrow mental handicap scene. Our recommendations lay great stress on the support to be given by the Primary Health Care Team and other back-up services. These services

are at present insufficient to give the support our model requires and additional money must be found to supplement them. This will be very expensive. There will also be costs involved in restructuring existing services to meet our management model.

367.   We could not estimate the resource implications of these essential activities with any degree of accuracy and we have therefore not made the attempt. But we feel that these additional costs should be brought to the Government's attention as a significant, though not immediately apparent, result of our recommendations. It would not be sensible to inject finance into residential care services only. There are other services which are equally important to mentally handicapped people and to their families and which are equally in need of expansion.

CHILDREN

368.   One of the results of an increase in spending on some of the important activities mentioned in the preceding paragraphs will be particularly noticeable in the residential care of mentally handicapped children. It is already clear that the White Paper overestimated the number of hospital places required for children in that there are already fewer children in hospital now than had been forecast in 1991. On the other hand it is also clear that the number of local authority children's places is grossly inadequate and the effect of this shortage of places may be made more acute by the measures now being taken to prevent children being admitted to hospital for purely social reasons. The increase in the number of more severely handicapped children in local authority care which we hope to see as a result of these measures will also lead to a need for more places and for better qualified staff trained according to our model.

369.   But the need for residential care often arises from lack of support to families, particularly when the child is very young. The development of such services as day care for young mentally handicapped children or temporary relief (short-term day or residential care) will take the pressure off families and reduce the demand for residential care outside the family. Fostering and adoption and better preventive measures will also reduce the demand for residential services. Thus expenditure in fringe areas reduces expenditure on direct residential care.

VOLUNTARY ORGANISATIONS

370.   Voluntary organisations play a very important part in the provision of residential services for mentally handicapped people. We have excluded the significant number of residential places which are provided by voluntary and private homes from our calculations of the need for staff in local authority residential services, but we are not implying any denigration of voluntary efforts. Our task is to look at the problems of the statutory services but we very much hope that the training of staff in voluntary and private homes will follow our model. Indeed many of the voluntary organisations such as the Spastics Society and Dr Barnado's have long been in the forefront of the development of residential care training. The voluntary sector has been involved in CSS schemes from the start; if our proposals make the schemes too

expensive for the voluntary bodies, the existing financial assistance for training provided by central Government to some of the voluntary societies will have to be extended.

SUMMING UP

371.   Whether our proposals can get off the ground depends on the attitude of the authorities who will have to provide the services and see that the staff who man them are properly trained. One of the most influential factors will be the availability of funds to enable health and social services authorities to finance the far reaching changes we recommend. In this Chapter we have tried to estimate the improvements which might be possible within the resources which are likely to be available to mental handicap over the next decade. We hope, of course, that the real growth in health and personal social services will be above the rates which we have used in our forecasts and if they are we can expect a more rapid achievement of our proposals.

372.   Having said that, mental handicap represents only a small percentage of total health and personal social services spending; less than 5% of revenue and less than 6% of capital expenditure in 1976/77. It is only a minute part of total Government expenditure and even a re-allocation of a tiny percentage of resources would have a dramatic impact on the possibilities for growth in the mental handicap services, which start from a very low baseline. We realise, however, that even if the money became available such growth would have to be adjusted to the practical limits set by the increases in other services, not necessarily provided by health and local social services authorities, upon which our recommendations depend.

CHAPTER 8– CONCLUSION

"Governments change, and the problems and the promises continue. There is no political capital to be made out of the needs of the mentally handicapped, and the goodwill and sincerity of those who try to bring about reform is unquestionable. Yet many of the problems seem to be intractable. We know some of the answers, just as we know some of the answers to the problems of war, pollution and famine; but the trick is in applying them."[30]

INTRODUCTION

373.   The recommendations in this Report arose out of the rights and needs of mentally handicapped people. In our Report we have touched on some of the problems of the current mental handicap services; in this final Chapter we restate these problems and explain why we think our recommendations provide the best solutions. We see our recommendations as the logical next step in the move towards community care but in this Chapter we also consider the consequences of *not* changing the training and organisation of mental handicap residential care staff.

374.   In the following paragraphs we have used quotations from various published documents. These quotations are not intended to be a representative sample of views on mental handicap services, but we think they help to illustrate some of the criticisms which have been made, and are still being made, about the way in which care is delivered. These comments provide proof that many of the major problems which were identified long ago still remain to be solved. *The views of those involved in mental handicap care support us in our belief that a policy of gradualism will never achieve a decent and dignified life for mentally handicapped people; what is needed is positive action and a political commitment to a major shift in priorities for expenditure.*

THE PROBLEM

375.   Our remit required us to consider how mental handicap residential care staff should be trained and organised so as to put into effect the new and developing policies on mental handicap residential care. Over the last 25 years attitudes to mental handicap have altered. New theories have led to changes in the mental handicap nursing syllabuses, new approaches in hospital care and the build-up of local authority residential services. But, despite the moves towards community care, the dichotomy of NHS and local authority services with separate staff training and organisational systems has remained. The old and unsuitable hospital buildings, the shortages of staff and money and sometimes also the old custodial models of care have all remained with us. As policies have changed many anomalies have begun to appear within the services. Some nurses have found it difficult to reconcile the new qualities required of them with the traditional perception of the role of the nurse, or to introduce the principles of community care into a large, old mental handicap hospital; increased expectations of what mentally handicapped people can achieve have led to dissatisfaction with the organisation and staffing levels of wards and homes which frequently reduce staff to the level of "custodians of the orifices". How can we transcend these physical difficulties and start to fulfil the mentally

handicapped individual's emotional needs? Kathleen Jones has written[30] of a "back ward":– "Nothing prepares the new (and often untrained) member of staff for the conditions on Ward 99. It is possible to get used to distressing sights and even to the continual deafening clamour which assails the ears. Even the regular staff did not get used to the smell, and all except one (who boasted of the fact) occasionally had to wear surgical masks when changing incontinent patients – a task which was to dominate the day's routine." Can we continue to defend a system which degrades both staff and residents in this way? Given that a vast increase in resources is unlikely to be made available and large numbers of staff cannot be recruited and trained overnight, what can be done now to improve the service to the resident? These are some of the questions which we had to answer.

OUR RECOMMENDATIONS

The Model

376. Our answer to the problems of mental handicap residential care is contained in our model of the way in which society should respond to the mentally handicapped individual. This model is based on respect for the individual and respect for those who care for him. The mentally handicapped person should have access to the full range of services and facilities available to the general public, and specialist services should be provided only where the general services cannot cope with a special need. But where special provisions are required they should offer a wide range of options in the three spheres of day, domiciliary and residential services. Mentally handicapped people in residential care should not be isolated from their neighbourhood or, more importantly, from their families. The staff who care for mentally handicapped residents should be compassionate and caring, but also professionally trained; their role should be to help each mentally handicapped person to develop mentally, physically and emotionally. Residents should live in small family-type groups sharing experiences informally with the staff, making their own decisions and taking necessary risks.

Care Staff Numbers

377. Mentally handicapped people in residential care need individual attention from highly trained staff. For the mentally handicapped adult or child every aspect of daily life offers an opportunity to learn self-help skills, but this is possible only if there are sufficient staff to make use of these opportunities. In addition to improved staff ratios mentally handicapped people need continuity of care from a semi-permanent group of familiar people. Staff, on the other hand need sufficient free time to get right away from the stresses of their work and should preferably not be expected to live on the premises. Calculations based on these considerations led us to recommend that the mental handicap residential services should have about 60,000 residential care staff of whom half should be qualified, the other half being in-service trained. This is almost double the current total, but our model and all our recommendations depend crucially on a great increase in the number of staff working in direct care. Maureen Oswin[29] has highlighted some of the consequences of relying on inadequate numbers of staff:– "When one nurse has to bathe nine heavy spastic children single-handed, standing for two hours in a hot, noisy bathroom,

140

she is left sweating and tired, with aching muscles and sore feet. At the end of an evening she has too little emotional or physical energy left even to pick up a child and cuddle him, let alone campaign for better conditions."

Training the Staff

378.   We believe that all people, mentally handicapped or not, share the same human needs. Further we believe that all mentally handicapped people in residential care (ie in homes and hospitals) have the same residential care needs as people in children's or old people's homes. We therefore recommend that all mental handicap residential care staff should share a common residential care training. Staff need to know both about mental handicap and about the needs of adults and children in residential communities; they also need practical skills in the specialist (mental handicap) and general (residential care) aspects of their work. Their training thus needs to include theoretical and practical elements. Different skills are required when working with children and this too must be recognised within the training. Bringing all these factors together we devised a new training system; this training had more in common with the courses for residential care staff promoted by the Central Council for Education and Training in Social Work than with the mental handicap nurse training of the General Nursing Councils. We therefore recommend that CCETSW should be asked to set up a special group to design and promote mental handicap residential care training within the framework (but with certain important modifications) of the Certificate in Social Service. Recruitment to the training courses would either be direct or through recruitment to a Trainee grade, with secondment to training within a specified maximum period.

379.   Apart from this qualifying training we saw a need for a less intellectually demanding but nonetheless thorough course of study and practice for the Basic Care Staff who would be assisting the qualified staff. In addition there should be refresher courses available to all staff to keep them abreast of current developments, and post-qualifying training for qualified staff to equip them for greater responsibilities. In particular the GNCs and CCETSW should collaborate to develop post-qualifying courses for staff to work with the most profoundly handicapped residents.

Organising the Staff

380.   The same arguments which led us to recommend a common training for health and social services staff also led us to recommend a unified career structure. Mental handicap should not be isolated from the mainstream of residential care and staff should be able to move not just between mental handicap hospitals and homes but also between children's and old people's homes, and homes for physically handicapped people. We therefore recommend a common career structure for mental handicap residential care staff in the NHS and local authorities.

381.   Within each residential Unit there should be residential care staff with differing levels of experience and skill. The responsibilities of caring for mentally handicapped residents require the skills of a qualified worker, but there is also a more practical role suitable for the in-service trained Basic Care

141

Worker. Trainees too have something to contribute to the workload. A proliferation of staff grades creates an institutional atmosphere and distances the staff from the residents and we therefore propose a "flat" career structure. The Head of each Unit should be at least a Qualified Care Worker but where greater skill and experience are called for the Unit Head should be an Advanced (Unit) Care Worker. Beyond the residential Unit there is a need for both professional advice and management responsibility. These two roles can sometimes lead to conflict and we therefore recommend a combined post of adviser/manager – Advanced (Management) Care Worker – to be responsible for a number of living units. On the next level the Senior Manager should plan and co-ordinate across service boundaries. Within the health service one of the Senior Managers or Advanced (Management) Care Staff would be nominated the Area Mental Handicap Services Officer, to represent mental handicap in Area planning. An Assistant Director would perform the same function in each local authority.

Financing Our Proposals

382. Inevitably our proposals would be expensive and our brief look at financial problems showed us that new funding arrangements would be required. We were forced – against all our beliefs – to resurrect the NHS/local authority dichotomy in terms of funding because the two services are financed in such different ways. In the NHS we found that an improvement in residential care staff/resident ratios could be achieved within our extrapolation of forecast expenditure if the resident population declined at the rate forecast by the White Paper. In the personal social services the low level of provision and the shortage of trained staff presented a less cheerful picture. We calculated that the extrapolated forecast revenue expenditure would pay for a considerable increase in residential care staff numbers but a special initiative would be required to get the new training off the ground. We therefore recommend that a special fund be established to meet some of the training costs.

SUMMING UP

"No Change"?

383. As a conclusion to our report we wish to re-affirm our belief that our recommendations are not only right for mental handicap but also necessary and inevitable. When considering our proposals it is important to bear in mind the alternatives. Many people may argue that no change is necessary and that the organisation and training of nurses and residential care staff will continue to evolve naturally. But the present evolution cannot continue indefinitely. In the NHS even if the Briggs Committee's proposals for a broadly based modular nurse training are not introduced there will be changes of some kind. In the local authorities, too, a policy of "no change" could not be sustained for long. Following White Paper policies local authority homes will admit an increasing number of the more severely handicapped people who are now in hospital, but the number of staff with any type of training in residential care will be increasing at a very slow rate. Without some special initiative it is most unlikely that our target of a 50% qualified/50% in-service trained workforce would ever be achieved in the local authorities.

384. *Without the changes which we have recommended mentally handi-capped people will continue to suffer the indignities to which countless surveys, enquiries and reports have drawn attention, and the care staff will be left to sort out as best they can the conflicting demands of theory and practice.* Having described some scenes from the life of one ward for 21 multiply handicapped children Maureen Oswin[29] asks:

"Which professionals could be held responsible for the deprived condi-tions in Ward 7, and the appalling loneliness of the children? There were no therapists working in the hospital; social workers never visited the ward; the doctors gave no guidance at ward level, apparently because they were engrossed with committee work and with out-patients; the nurses appeared to be fighting a losing battle because of shortages of staff, and their goodwill and kindness was being dissipated by the poor conditions and lack of support."

Even if only one ward like this exists it is still one ward too many.

385. For decades we have known how to put right the appalling conditions to which mentally handicapped people and those who care for them are subjected, and for decades we have allowed those same conditions to survive. Mental handicap services have been high on the list of priorities in recent years and have grown faster than other areas in the health and personal social services. But incremental growth is not enough. Minor improvements in man-power or staff training cannot alter the character of services which have suffered from years of shortages and neglect. *If action is not taken now to ensure that the principles of community care can be put into practice in every mental handicap hospital and home, then another Committee of Enquiry will be required in 10 or 20 years' time to look at the problems of mental handicap care staff.*

386. We are confident that our arguments will be sufficient to convince the Government that action must be taken now. Throughout our work we have been aware of the need to be practical; mentally handicapped people and those who care for them have no need of utopian visions. *Our recommen-dations call for more resources for mental handicap, but the implementation of our proposals would require only a tiny shift in priorities for public spending. We trust that the Government will find the determination to make that shift.*

LIST OF MAIN RECOMMENDATIONS

The recommendations which follow are dependent upon the introduction of our model of care as described in Chapter 3. This model is based on the three principles of (a) normal patterns of life; (b) respect for individuality; and (c) the provision of help from the neighbourhood community and from professional services. Our model also calls for increased involvement with mentally handicapped people and those who care for them from a wide range of support services. In particular the Primary Health Care Team will need to play a larger role in supporting families with a mentally handicapped member and the various specialists – psychiatrists, psychologists, remedial professions, paediatricians and other medical specialists – should be willing to extend their services to mentally handicapped people.

Manpower

1. Once our model of care has been put into effect its manpower implications should be subject to continuing monitoring and evaluation (para 169).

2. There should be an approximate doubling of mental handicap residential care staff (ie those in direct contact with residents) (para 184).

3. Health and social services authorities should press ahead towards the staffing target of 60,000 direct residential care staff as fast as their finances will allow (para 185).

4. Responsibility for the day-time activities of adult residents during the week should be with staff trained to teach mentally handicapped people (para 195).

5. If there is to be any special drive on recruitment, expenditure should be focussed on Trainees (para 205).

Staff Training

6. Mental handicap residential care staff in the health and social services should receive a common training (para 218).

7. Mental handicap residential care workers should undertake a training which will provide for both the generic residential care and the unique mental handicap care components of their work. These two elements should be covered in both theoretical and practical work (para 221).

8. As part of the qualifying training there should be separate modules for those who will work with adults and those who will work with children and adolescents. These modules should include both practical and theoretical elements (para 222).

9. Qualifying training should be fulltime, with equal periods of theory and practice (para 223).

10. Recruitment to the qualifying training should be:

 a. through the Trainee grade, with secondment after a maximum of two years, or

 b. by direct recruitment to the training course (para 224).

144

11.   Even during the pre-secondment period, the learning needs of Trainees should be paramount (para 225).

12.   The training of mental handicap residential care staff should be placed within the main stream of residential care, under the aegis of CCETSW and following the broad framework of the Certificate in Social Service, but with the essential additional provisions which we have described (para 241).

13.   CSS certificates should state clearly the specialism studied (para 244).

14.   CQSW-trained staff who wish to work in the residential care of mentally handicapped people should have had specialist training equivalent to the mental handicap special unit on CSS (para 245).

15.   CCETSW should make the necessary modifications to the CSS which should become the training for qualified mental handicap care staff (para 246).

16.   All Trainees should have experience of small group living in some shape or form (para 247).

17.   The special group within CCETSW should consider the problem of the effects of maldistribution of mental handicap residential care establishments on the provision of practice placements, and issue advice on the subject to course planners (para 248).

18.   Decisions on the use of any spare capacity in the nurse training schools should be left to individual AHAs (para 251).

19.   Employing authorities should designate a training organiser or some other person to ensure that each member of staff is involved in an on-going training programme suited to his needs (para 252).

20.   Every member of staff should receive formal induction training and should be encouraged to attend refresher or specialist training courses (para 254).

21.   Employing authorities should provide formal in-service training of at least two weeks' equivalent in each year for all Basic Care staff (para 255).

22.   Mentally handicapped people who require general, paediatric or psychiatric hospital treatment should be cared for in hospital by general, sick children's or psychiatric nurses and that the training of these nurses should include an understanding of mental handicap (para 257).

23.   The General Nursing Councils and the Central Council for Education and Training in Social Work should collaborate on the development of post-qualifying courses for Qualified Care staff and general, psychiatric and sick children's nurses working with very severely handicapped residents (para 258).

24.   Post-qualifying courses should be available for all staff at the Qualified Care Worker grade and above (para 259).

25.   Health and education authorities should jointly consider the question of transferability of teaching qualifications (para 263).

26.   All new mental handicap residential care CSS schemes should include preliminary courses for teaching staff; these courses should be extended to include instruction in our model of care (para 264).

145

27. Health, social services and education authorities should come together in local committees to plan the introduction of the new training (para 267).

28. All existing staff should attend seminars and study days to learn about our Report and discuss its implications for them (para 270).

29. Employing authorities and training bodies should re-examine their existing courses for senior staff to ensure that in the light of our Report, senior staff are given the opportunity to explore the new perspectives on mental handicap residential care (para 271).

Organisation and Management

30. There should not be a separate new mental handicap residential caring profession (para 278).

31. Entry to the qualifying training should be at the age of 18, since we do not wish to see anyone taking on the responsibilities of a qualified staff member before the age of 20 (para 286).

32. Individual employing authorities should be allowed to decide on the grading of each post of Unit Head, but all Unit Heads must be qualified and experienced mental handicap residential care staff. Heads of children's Units, like other qualified staff working in these Units, must have taken the children's module in their training (para 289).

33. Advanced (Management) Care staff should have dual responsibility for both management and the quality of service (para 291).

34. There should be a ratio of approximately 1:1 for Basic Care staff to Qualified staff (up to and including Senior Manager). Within Units there should be a ratio of 1 Qualified Care Worker to 1.3 Basic Care staff and 1 Advanced (Unit) Care Worker to 2.6 Qualified Care staff thus 50% of the workforce should be qualified and 50% in-service trained (para 296).

35. Each health authority should appoint an Area Mental Handicap Services Officer, accountable directly to the Area Health Authority, to represent mental handicap at the higher levels of NHS management (para 301).

36. Employers and professional associations concerned should consider the problem of disciplinary powers and agree on a system of professional discipline at the earliest possible opportunity (para 322).

37. The negotiating bodies should try and work towards a unified salary structure and common conditions of service for mental handicap residential care staff in the NHS and social services departments at the earliest possible opportunity (para 323).

38. Each employing authority should set a date after which it will not recruit unqualified or unsuitably qualified staff to the Qualified Care Worker grade and above (para 325).

39. At the end of an interim period all staff in Qualified Care Worker posts and above should be accepted as "qualified staff". During and after the interim period these existing staff should be awarded the pay, terms and

146

conditions of service and prospects appropriate to qualified staff. After the interim period, recognition of qualifications should be limited to the following:–

CSS (our proposed mental handicap residential care version only),

RNMS (RMND in Scotland),

SEN (MS) (Enrolled Nurse in Scotland),

CQSW (only if sufficient specialist work has been undertaken),

Specific CSS/CQSW courses which replaced CRSW, CRCCYP or SCRCCYP courses (para 326).

40.   After the interim period, recruitment and promotion to any qualified grade should be limited to those with a recognised qualification (para 327).

41.   A National Staff Commission should be established to supervise the introduction of our proposals and to adjudicate on any complaints from existing staff (para 333).

42.   Existing staff should be treated generously in the implementation of our structure (para 333).

43.   Direct care staff should be given a clothing allowance and permitted to choose whether to wear a uniform/overall (para 338).

44.   Any mental handicap nurse who prefers to remain in nursing should be offered a place on one of the shortened courses for nurses wishing to transfer from one part of the Register or Roll to another (para 339).

45.   The National Staff Commission should be asked to consider problems of pay and conditions of service at the earliest opportunity and to ensure that no existing member of staff will lose by our recommendations (para 340).

Finance and Priorities

46.   The "Sheffield Method" staff ratios should be introduced nationally as quickly as possible (para 355).

47.   A central fund should be established to underwrite certain key aspects of staff training (para 362).

1. PERSONAL STATEMENT BY BETTY NICOLAS

GENERAL NURSING COUNCIL FOR ENGLAND AND WALES

1. As Education Officer to the General Nursing Council for England and Wales with special responsibility for mental subnormality nurse training and in view of the fact that the Report has special implications for the Council, I think it important to make a personal statement and am grateful for the opportunity to include this in the Report.

2. As an independent member of the Jay Committee, I support the philosophy and the model of care which are the basis of the Committee's Report and which lead logically to the conclusions for training which are described in the Report.

3. In contributing to the deliberations of the Committee to the Report, I have tried at all times to act as an expert witness with a special knowledge of mental subnormality nurse training and of the policies of the General Nursing Council and to keep the Committee informed of current General Nursing Council thinking and policy.

4. The Council gave evidence both written (published) and oral to the Committee in which it stated its then present commitment to the preparation of nurses for the care of the mentally subnormal.

5. My personal acceptance of the Report as a member of the Jay Committee in no way commits the Mental Nurses Committee or the Council to any particular views or course of action.

Betty Nicolas.

2. PERSONAL STATEMENT BY PRISCILLA YOUNG, DIRECTOR, CENTRAL COUNCIL FOR EDUCATION AND TRAINING IN SOCIAL WORK

1. The recommendations contained in the Jay Committee's Report have important implications for the work of CCETSW, the training body of which I am currently the Director. As I have been a member of the Committee, I think it important to include in the Report a personal statement of my position, and I am grateful to the Chairman and other members for permitting me to do this.

2. I give unqualified support to the philosophy which we have set out in the Report, and I find the ideas on which the model of care are based entirely convincing. If one accepts these approaches to the residential care of mentally handicapped people, the logic of the recommendations regarding the general nature of training provision seems to me inescapable.

3. However, the Committee has also made some quite specific recommendations which, if accepted, would have significant effects, not only upon the work of CCETSW but also its staffing and structure. The Committee has studied in detail the scheme of training leading to the award of the Certificate in Social Service and has expressed views about the way in which this particular form of training should be modified and developed to meet the needs of residential care staff in both health service units and local authority and voluntary sector provision for mentally handicapped people.

4. In discussions on these matters I have thought it proper to act more as an "expert witness" than as a member of the Committee, and I have endeavoured to provide full information about existing training programmes, and the current policies of CCETSW, in order to help the Committee reach its decisions.

I have not participated in the exact formulation of recommendations which have direct implications for CCETSW, and my membership of the Jay Committee should in no sense be taken as committing the Council to any specific views or to a particular course of action.

Nevertheless, I can state with confidence that both the Council and its staff wish to do everything in their power to ensure the proper development of training for those staff working with mentally handicapped people, for whom the Council has training responsibilities.

Priscilla H. F. Young.

NOTE OF DISSENT BY MR NICK BOSANQUET

I accept fully the philosophy and the model of care set out in the Report. There has been an increasing amount of agreement about the desirable pattern of community care for the mentally handicapped and there will probably be a welcome for the Report's general philosophy. My worry is about the difficulties in the way of turning these aspirations into reality. Of course, the Committee has given a great deal of thought to these problems and has taken them into account in framing its recommendations. On balance, however, I do not think it has gone far enough. We are making our recommendations against a good deal of experience. On past experience community care was slow to grow even where it involved little direct co-operation between the NHS and local authorities. Now we are suggesting a much greater degree of co-operation even though the main responsibility would still be with the NHS in the first few years. I am concerned about the halting response of many local authorities even when fewer demands were put on them. I am also doubtful whether we have allowed enough for a second major difficulty – the fears and worries of many staff in the mental handicap hospitals. Of course, the Committee is deeply concerned about these but I do not think that the safeguards proposed are adequate. These difficulties, in my view, will be great enough to ensure that little progress is made with the new training if it is organised and financed in the ways suggested in the Report.

We are all agreed on the very great need for change in patterns of care, and of training. The majority of staff working in the hospitals, to judge from our own survey, want to see change. Certainly, the shortage of staff is one reason for the lack of progress towards a 'social' model of care: but the balance of evidence from our own survey and from NDG Reports as well as from the earlier survey by Kathleen Jones does suggest a considerable need for change in attitudes for greater teamwork and for a more informed and somewhat more optimistic approach to the care of mentally handicapped people. Of course more training alone will not be enough. We need more small units in the community. These will give residents a much better chance of working outside, of some privacy at home and of keeping in touch with their relatives. It will also give more hope of individual help and attention to the severely handicapped. A changed pattern of training with some promise of security for years to come is, however, an essential complement to these general changes. It is mainly because change is so much needed and could mean so much in terms of opportunities for the mentally handicapped that we have to be realistic about facing the difficulties.

There is still a very long way to go towards even a minimal amount of service in the community, particularly for the severely handicapped. It is still very uncommon to find severely handicapped people being cared for in small units in the community. As our own survey shows the great majority of residents in local authority hostels are more lightly handicapped; most severely handicapped people in long-term residential care are in hospitals. The challenge of caring for severely handicapped people in a community setting has been met in only a very few places. There is still a considerable amount of disbelief and anxiety to be overcome on this point.

150

There is also scepticism about whether all local authorities want to do the job, even among those who accept that they can and should do it. For more than 10 years local authorities were asked and urged to build some residential places for the mentally handicapped. Even now, however, there is a substantial minority of local authorities which have not taken many steps towards doing this. There are some who have no residential places of their own for children. There are even some who have no places at all, either for adults or for children although under present plans this group will virtually disappear by 1980. Now the Committee is asking that local authorities should undertake a more ambitious staff training programme. It is hardly surprising in the light of the past record that there should be some scepticism about whether local authorities can do this.

The doubts are increased by the enormous size of the task which local government faces in training for the social services generally. It is well known that the level of training is low among residential care staff. In one report by CCETSW it was estimated that only 4% of residential care staff had had any specific training in residential care. The general level is low even though our own survey shows the position to be considerably better for mental handicap staff. The training effort is still heavily biased towards field staff. There are also strong disincentives on any one authority to do more training. The Authority pays most of the costs, but the benefits often may accrue elsewhere as staff move. The Committee is recommending an increased programme of training for residential staff working with the mentally handicapped. Of course there may be some special assistance, but even as recommended this will not cover all the costs. The part of the new programme which affects local authorities will have to be fitted into a social services budget for training which is small and unlikely, except through special arrangements, to grow much larger. It has also to be fitted within the even smaller budget for the training of residential care staff. Even with special help I doubt whether local government can take the amount of initiative asked for in the Report. Special help to probation and child care training in the 1960's are mentioned as precedents for the scheme of special financial help suggested in the Report. But the overall financial situation of local government was then much more favourable and we did not have social service departments within which, in my experience, all claims have to be weighed finely against the claims of competing groups.

The other main area of difficulty lies with the views of staff working in hospitals. Some of them think that the current prospectus for community care is far too optimistic. They accept that change is required, but they also feel extremely concerned about a possible loss of identity, commitment and professional standing in the event of change. Like the Committee, I take these fears very seriously but I do not think we have allayed them. It is unthinkable that any solution could be imposed on staff without their consent. We all agree that staff amount to perhaps the most important resource which the services can have. Even now most of the trained staff working not just in the hospitals but also in the local authority hostels, have received their training in the hospitals and this will continue for some time to come. We have to make

151

recommendations which will mean movement towards the new model of care but they also must be recommendations which are broadly acceptable to staff and which go some way towards allaying fears. The Committee has aimed to do this. In many respects it has succeeded but in my view there are still some vital gaps.

The Committee's proposals cover the relationship of the new training to other forms of social service training, a pattern of qualification, the role of CCETSW and special financial arrangements. The Report is essentially recommending that most training should be done within the CSS framework but with a degree of specialisation. The qualification is to have the same basis as other forms of social service qualification. CCETSW is to be asked to set up a special committee to oversee the training and to give some special degree of administrative backing. Finally, some special arrangements are being suggested for financing the training. These proposals can only work if local and health authorities themselves are prepared to take a considerable degree of initiative and so long as there is confidence about the long-term development and standing of the CSS qualification. If there is serious doubt about the ability particularly of local government to take the initiative and if there is a great deal of worry about the CSS qualification, then there is little in these proposals to ensure movement ahead. These measures might well work in a climate or context which was basically favourable – but they are unlikely to be enough to make up for the likely inertia of local authorities and the anxieties of staff. In my view we need an initiative of a different kind if the new model of training is to have a full chance of success.

I would propose, therefore, a separate training council established by legislation and which would administer a new pattern of statutory qualifications. The content of the courses and the pattern of different qualifications would be much as set out in the Report. There is no reason why there should not be a considerable degree of local initiative in the curriculum as is planned for the CSS course. The membership of the training council would cover both the local authority and the health services. The Council would organise courses centred both on existing schools of nursing and on a number of Colleges of Further Education. It might also organise some courses based in universities and polytechnics. The new basic qualification might be called a Certificate in Mental Handicap, and there would also be opportunities to specialise in particular areas of care. The statutory body would be independent of CCETSW but the two councils would obviously want to develop a close working relationship. The new training, in so far as it involved the NHS, would be financed by central government in roughly the same way as is nurse training at present. Those courses and placements which involved local authorities would be financed by special supplement to joint funding, at least for the first years. In general therefore all finance, including the salaries of trainees, would in one way or another be underwritten by central funding.

It would obviously be very important for the new training to be planned in close association with CCETSW. In the very long term it might be possible to relate the new statutory body even more closely with CCETSW. It is widely believed that the new training should not and could not stay within the framework of nurse training particularly after the 'Briggs' training begins: but there is a strong body of support in the Committee and outside that the training for all staff should go to CCETSW. Under my proposal there would be room for close consultation between the new body, CCETSW and the GNC.

It will be argued that such a proposal for a separate training council would be divisive and in the words of the Report would "perpetuate the dogma of special services and special staff". But I share some of the doubt that has grown up in the last few years about the concept of generic training. There is a growing view that there ought to be more specialisation within a common philosophy of caring and a common core of knowledge about people. The Committee's own proposals represent some move towards specialisation. My proposal represents an attempt to create a greater identity for the training and it certainly does aspire to attract and train people specifically for work with the mentally handicapped. The proposal would mean a chance for a different model of training to that which has resulted from the Seebohm Report.

In my view, community care will grow naturally as the new training develops and the new services expand. The danger is that in our intention to serve community care we will in fact take steps which will impede its natural growth locally. I believe that under my proposals there is more likely to be a substantial number of people in 10 years' time trained for a new social model of care than there will be under the Committee's proposals. It would be folly to jeopardise the reality of the new training and the new philosophy mainly because of what I would regard as the less important issues of the administrative arrangements for it and the labels.

NOTE OF DISSENT BY DR DEREK RICKS

Firstly, I want to emphasise my wholehearted support of the majority of recommendations made by my colleagues on the Committee.

The issue on which I differ, and one which has been my major concern throughout our discussions, is whether our recommendations adequately safeguard the care of the severely handicapped such as the very dependent or disturbed. I do not think they do. Although small in number the quality of their care is crucial to the standards set for the residential service future staff will provide. Currently such profoundly handicapped people are described as needing hospital care, a term which in reality relates less to their need for, or likelihood of receiving, specialised medical or nursing care than to their unacceptability to residential agencies outside hospital. In most cases the basic criteria for hospital admission, as staff there well know, is that they alone are prepared or obliged to cope with the prospective resident. This, agreed by all members of the Committee, is a totally unsatisfactory state of affairs. To remedy it requires that the most handicapped are incorporated into our model of care which means that the recruitment and training of staff we suggest equips them to deal with *all* the handicapped. I do not believe that this can be achieved by training organised by CCETSW.

From the onset of our deliberations I have drawn attention to this crucial issue and had hoped that persuading colleagues of the need for, and the role of the NHS back-up service would both cater for the needs of this group and overcome the very real anxieties any staff will face in their care. I feel an NHS back-up service to be fundamental to the feasibility of our recommendations and I think it has been given inadequate emphasis in the final form of our Report. But if the back-up service is to function as recommended, if it is to avoid becoming a dumping ground for the unmanageable elsewhere, then its task must be remedial and defined and its residential commitment must be limited to the time needed to solve the particular problem preventing the handicapped person living within the array of residential units supported by that service. Its obligation is to establish treatment programmes which work in the handicapped person's home to the satisfaction of those residential staff (or his parents) caring for him. Similarly, and equally important, it is the obligation of that caring staff to accept his return which means they must themselves be prepared and able to use advice and thus equipped to cope. Otherwise the support services will soon be swamped.

Accepting that the issue fundamental to my viewpoint was how to ensure as far as possible this coping capacity in residential staff I thought at length over my daily working experience. I tried to think very carefully why nurses in hospital usually do cope with the most difficult handicapped people while (with some notable exceptions) staff in the community rarely do. There are of course a whole variety of reasons, some of them quite negative. One of them, not unimportant, is that nursing staff like some parents have no option. Other reasons relate to practices and a system of care broadly termed 'custodial' and which the Report if implemented will go far to remedy – much, I feel sure, to the relief of staff who are currently compelled to implement that system. But an important positive reason, I feel, is that those who cope sympathetically with the permanent care of the most severely handicapped are committed specifically to the care of the *handicapped* in the way that the best nurses are now. Certainly all those people whom I have learned to respect as coping devotedly and constructively with such a burden of care have joined whatever part of the service they are in, community or hospital, because they wanted to care solely for the handicapped. I am convinced this quality of specific commitment is fundamental. Without it those among the handicapped most needing care, and those families most needing relief, will not be accommodated within the excellent system of staffed units we are advocating. I believe the best way, perhaps the only way, to secure this quality of commitment is for the staff recruited to have a separate professional identity and therefore their own training body. I would hope that such a step would be most likely to retain and promote a professional pride ensuring that the working perspective of such staff automatically reached to the most handicapped and would scorn to restrict itself to the care of the more able and less demanding.

I accept that advocating a separate profession caring for the handicapped conflicts with the conviction, which I greatly respect, of my colleagues that those who care for the mentally handicapped should be trained within the main stream of residential care. I appreciate and have been impressed by their humane, compassionate arguments. I further accept that my own viewpoint in its effort to secure what I feel to be a fundamental safeguard, could be construed as segregating the handicapped and supporting a system of care which denies them access to social experiences which the non-handicapped enjoy. I do not accept that this is a necessary consequence of my recommendations. Indeed, what impresses me about many staff committed solely to the care of the handicapped is their readiness to strive for small gains, and their acceptance of slow progress which sustains their enthusiasm to push wider the social horizons of those they care for. I think that these striving attitudes are part of their commitment which is fostered, not hindered, by their working familiarity with even the most handicapped. However, I strongly endorse the Committee's view that experience of residential care of the non-handicapped is an imperative component of training particularly for the care of handicapped children. This is in no way incompatible with the training of a separate caring profession.

Having reached the conclusion that I should advocate a separate caring profession the question then arose whether the members of that profession should be nurses. Certainly in the care of the most severely handicapped distinctive skills are needed to remedy, or at least contain, their frequent physiological and psychiatric peculiarities. But appreciating that many such distinctive needs are consistently and adequately met by parents I do not feel this is a valid argument. If, at any given time, such needs are urgent or severe they would be met either by general medical or educational services (though this often presents major problems as many parents know) or by the staff of a back-up service.

There were two reasons why I did not feel able to press that the separate profession should consist of specialised nurses. The first was that as nurses they could not avail themselves of the simpler administrative structure advocated by this Committee. The second was that a separate non-nursing caring

155

profession would enjoy autonomy and must accept responsibility for the care of its residents because it would have a different working relationship with doctors and paramedical staff. The expertise of these latter professional groups would be provided on request through the back-up service: this would enable its practitioners to concentrate their clinical skills on the supervision and management of handicapped people referred to them for specific reasons rather than as an open-ended, clinically undefined residential commitment. At the same time those caring staff, either now or in the future, whose primary interest is in working as nurses within a team to investigate and remedy clinical problems in the handicapped wherever they live will find a fulfilling role in the back-up service.

By distinguishing between care staff responsible for residential provisions for all the handicapped and nursing staff I would hope to concentrate and contain appropriately skills of the latter and facilitate the social emphasis of care in the former. By this means each group has the opportunity to work in a way not only more fulfilling to themselves but to the welfare and home environment of all the handicapped. To make this feasible and to ensure that the substance of the Committee's proposals are implemented requires, in my opinion, that we have a staff caring with support for the full spectrum of the handicapped. A level of commitment is needed for this which I feel requires the independence and status of a separate qualified profession.

MINORITY REPORT BY MR D O WILLIAMS

1.   The Committee of Enquiry was established by the Secretary of State for Social Services in 1975 in order to review the work and training of nurses and local authority care staff who care for the mentally handicapped, taking full account of the Briggs recommendation that a "new caring profession . . . should emerge gradually", of the existing roles and aims of nurses and residential care staff, and of the need to make the best use of available skills and experience.

2.   The need for change has been recognised and accepted by those working with the mentally handicapped and involved in their direct day-to-day care. It is vital, however, that change must build upon the strengths and assets of the existing service as well as looking to new ideas and methods. It is vital, also, that the recommendations of the Committee will enjoy the confidence and support of the existing profession. While I agree with much of the majority report, it is my view that some of the main recommendations will be unacceptable to those who provide most of the existing care for the mentally handicapped. I am, therefore, unable to support those particular recommendations outlined below for the reasons given. In essence, I believe that the Committee has failed to give due weight to the strengths of the present service and that this failure will undermine the confidence and morale of the dedicated staff at present responsible for the day-to-day care of the mentally handicapped.

3.   Let me say at once that I agree with my colleagues that in order to improve the quality of care for the mentally handicapped there must be a new approach which will ensure that, regardless of where or by whom the care is provided, there must be as normal a life-style as possible. I accept that this involves the mentally handicapped remaining in their own homes wherever possible – with all the resource allocation that this entails, with fostering whenever possible, and with admission to residential accommodation resorted to only when other alternatives have been exhausted.

4.   The two substantial questions on which I depart from the majority are:—

(i)   who should provide and administer the residential services, and

(ii)   what form of training and qualification the staff require.

The Residential Services

5.   The majority Report reflects the view expressed in the White Paper that a substantial part of the care of the mentally handicapped should be transferred from the NHS to the local authority social services. I have never accepted this view; furthermore, I fear that the effect of the Committee's Report will not simply be to support but to accelerate this movement towards local authority care. I believe that small family units in the community can be provided by the NHS, but perhaps more importantly, I do not share the confidence of my colleagues in the social services as potential providers of both the services and accommodation required. Mental handicap is not necessarily considered by

157

the local electorate to be a high priority and the extent of social provision will, eventually, be determined by ratepayers' priorities. This was amply demonstrated prior to 1948 when the NHS took over the administration of local authority hospitals which were showing signs of chronic under-financing and the NHS was seen, quite rightly, to be the only way of providing the necessary resources to raise standards to a national level of acceptability. Mental handicap had proved to be the lowest of priorities for the majority of local authorities. To accelerate the transfer of residential care from the NHS to social services is, in my view, to risk reverting to that form of inconsistent and inadequate provision for the mentally handicapped. It is my view that a unified service, which would include responsibility for existing local authority provision, should be administered by the NHS.

6. The 1971 White Paper was critical of the level of provision made by local authorities for the mentally handicapped and today I can see very little evidence to suggest that attitudes and priorities have changed enough everywhere. Certainly, there is nowhere near enough evidence for me to accept with confidence that the proposals of the majority would be implemented as they envisage. Representatives of the local authority associations, appearing before the Committee, told us that they "could do a better job" given the same resources as the NHS. I treat this assertion with considerable scepticism given their general lack of experience and expertise in providing for the mentally handicapped. A few local authorities have failed lamentably to make the necessary provisions for the mentally handicapped and mentally ill under the 1959 Mental Health Act, the Health Services and Public Health Act 1968 and other relevant legislation – for example, in terms of providing hostel accommodation for the mentally ill as an alternative to hospital. There is strong evidence of a marked reluctance on the part of some of these local authorities to provide similar residential accommodation for the mentally handicapped in the community. If this is the case under the minimum provisions required of them at present, how much worse is the situation likely to be if the whole range of mental handicap services were entrusted to them?

7. Of serious concern also is the appallingly low level of qualified staff working in social services. Only a very small proportion are trained, and greater access to training is a major question at the present time. There can be little prospect of improvement in the next few years and the future of any social service based mental handicap service would therefore seem to be very uncertain.

8. In strong contrast to what I consider to be the poor record of local authorities in community based residential care, the NHS has brought about many wide-ranging improvements in the care of both the mentally handicapped and mentally ill. It has kept abreast of current thinking and developments in this country and abroad. Ward numbers have been dramatically reduced, partly by dividing and sub-dividing old wards but also by building new hospitals. Attitudes are rapidly changing from custodial care to dynamic therapeutic programmes, matched by improved and better training of nurses arising from changing the RMPA to the regularly reviewed and up-dated RNMS. The whole point is that the NHS is geared to introducing those

changes, in the majority Report, which are designed to improve the quality of care, and it has already been shown to have the flexibility needed to absorb new ideas easily.

9. Furthermore, those who advocate a transfer of the service have not taken sufficient account, in my view, of the enormous upheaval caused by such a move, and which would not be in the interests of the handicapped. In the foreseeable future responsibility for the service would be divided between the NHS and the local authority which would create problems both of organisation and of allocating those in need of care.

10. A complex but fragmented new structure, involving a large number of highly qualified professional and administrative staff would be needed and many difficulties would occur of the type currently experienced in joint financing. To recommend a structure which would extend this type of divided responsibility is to build in more problems than we are trying to resolve.

11. I also believe that the allocation of those in need of care in such a situation of joint responsibility would inevitably lead to streaming, with those most severely handicapped receiving less favourable treatment. This would not happen in a properly integrated and unified service which could provide comprehensive facilities for all levels of handicap.

Professional Training

12. It is my unequivocal view that the most appropriate form of training for those working with the mentally handicapped should continue to be the 3-year training leading to a professional nursing qualification. The length of training should not be reduced, although the syllabus should be changed so as to lay more emphasis on the social aspects of care, on the basis recommended in chapter 4 of the Briggs Report. It should also change, in common with other nurse training, as recommended by Briggs.

13. The RNMS should, therefore, be regarded as the necessary and appropriate qualification for those caring for the mentally handicapped both in the hospital and the local authority residential home or unit. Accordingly I do not accept that there is a role for CCETSW as the majority Report recommends. The training envisaged under the Central Council would not lead in any sense to a professional qualification. Without a professional qualification, there is no profession. The majority Report runs the unjustifiable risk, in my view, of creating a diluted and generic certificate, involving a varying period of training, instead of allowing a new caring profession to evolve as originally recommended by the Briggs Report. Those employed in caring for the mentally handicapped in future would not have the status currently enjoyed by nurses, and this would be a severe blow to the morale of those whose devotion, in often difficult and unpleasant circumstances, now provides that care.

14. The Committee's proposal is for the care worker to receive the Certificate in Social Service (CSS) training – a training of recent origin, available to most people employed in the social services but not a *professional* qualification. It is not specifically designed for staff in residential work, nor for those working with the mentally handicapped. Even with the inclusion of a module

for mental handicap, it is of shorter duration than the RNMS course. It concerns itself with local needs rather than with preparing an individual for full professional development, hence the comments in the majority report about the need to ensure that those working with mentally handicapped children should be experienced in children's work. In contrast, the specialised RNMS qualification has proved its worth in practice, demonstrated its flexibility in responding to change over the years, and has provided a viable career structure for caring staff. Further developed as recommended by Briggs, RNMS training does and will provide the best guarantee of proper care standards for the mentally handicapped.

Conclusion

15. The Committee has made a tremendous effort to establish a new caring profession, but in my view it had failed in its task. The new-type care worker would not be an acceptable successor to the nurse and as I believe that the standard of care would be lowered, I regret I cannot be a signatory to the main Report.

EVIDENCE QUESTIONNAIRE

This questionnaire was issued to all health and social services authorities, other relevant statutory and voluntary bodies and to individuals and organisations who requested copies.

COMMITTEE OF ENQUIRY INTO NURSING AND CARE OF THE MENTALLY HANDICAPPED

EVIDENCE FOR THE COMMITTEE

The Terms of Reference are

"To consider recommendation 74 of the Report of the Committee on Nursing (Briggs Committee), in particular to enquire into the nursing and care of the mentally handicapped in the light of developing policies, to examine the roles and aims of nurses and residential care staff required by the health and personal social services for the care of mentally handicapped adults and children; the inter-relationship between them and other health and personal social services staff; how existing staff can best fulfil these roles and aims; in the interest of making the best use of available skills and experience, the possibilities of the career movement of staff from one sector or category to another; the implications for recruitment and training; and to make recommendations."

The purpose of the attached questions is to indicate areas which the Committee feels are most important, and to help to provide a logically sequenced framework within which the Committee can consider the views of witnesses.

We realise that many witnesses will wish to answer only certain questions; some may want to extend into additional areas; others may wish simply to make a personal statement. This will be accepted providing comments fall within the general terms of reference of the Committee.

To help witnesses a summary of Chapter 3 of the White Paper "Better Services for the Mentally Handicapped" is attached.

Replies should be sent to the Secretary, Mr D Dufton, Room C405, Alexander Fleming House, Elephant and Castle, London SE1 6BY, as soon as possible and not later than 1 March 1976.

QUESTIONNAIRE

A. SERVICES

In June 1971 the White Paper "Better Services for the Mentally Handicapped" reviewed existing services for the mentally handicapped and in Chapter 3 spelled out the main principles on which current thinking about mental handicap was based. In February 1975 the philosophy and general approach of the White Paper were reaffirmed by the Secretary of State for Social Services. On 1 April 1971 Local Education Authorities assumed responsibility for the education of mentally handicapped children. In Scotland the relevant memorandum is "Services for the Mentally Handicapped" published jointly by the Scottish Home and Health Department and the Scottish Education Department in April 1972 and the Scottish Education Act 1974.

1. What suggestion would you make within this policy for the future development of services for the care of mentally handicapped people and their families?
2. Where would you place your priorities?
3. Are there any other principles that you would like to see emphasised and considered?

4.   Would you give your views on the alternative residential day care and other domiciliary services which would be required to implement and sustain a policy of caring for mentally handicapped people in the community.

B.   TASKS AND ROLES

In this section the Committee is interested in your views about the work which must be undertaken by many different people in order to give mentally handicapped individuals and their families a good service. In the following questions this work is referred to as "task".

It is also interested in the ways in which decisions are made about the care given and what responsibility for these decisions lies within the power of staff at various levels and in various disciplines and in the inter-relationships between the wide range of people who may be offering the care. These concepts are implicit in the word "role".

Some of the questions will refer to work now undertaken. Some will ask your views about what should happen in the future.

5.   TASKS

(a)   Can you describe the major tasks involved in providing services for mentally handicapped people and their families *currently* being performed by:

    (i)   Nurses working within the NHS?

    (ii)   Residential care staff in local authorities, hospital services and/or voluntary agencies?

    (iii)   Other personnel eg social workers, doctors, health visitors, psychologists, remedial professions, teachers, day care staff, domestic staff etc?

    (iv)   Parents and families?

(b)   Do some of these tasks have particular importance and relevance in the care of certain people, for instance a profoundly handicapped child; an adult with severe physical disabilities; a mildly handicapped adult; a mentally handicapped offender?

(c)   Which of these tasks have particular importance in supporting mentally handicapped people in their own homes?

(d)   Are any of these tasks currently being carried out in the homes of mentally handicapped people by staff based in residential units (hospitals and local authority homes)?

6.   What constraints operate at present on the tasks you have described above?

7.   What development and changes would you like to see in the tasks you have described above?

8.   ROLES

(a)   What are the major roles *currently* being performed by:

    (i)   Nurses working within the NHS?

    (ii)   Residential care staff in local authorities, hospital services and/or voluntary agencies?

    (iii)   Other personnel eg social workers, doctors, health visitors, psychologists, remedial professions, teachers, day care staff, domestic staff etc?

    (iv)   Parents and families?

162

(b)   What are the relationships between the roles of staff at various levels in residential services?

(c)   What are the relationships between the roles of staff in residential services, other health and social services staff, teachers, parents and families?

(d)   Is the concept of "overall clinical responsibility" for "patients" a useful or necessary one?

9.   What constraints operate at present on the performance of the roles you have described above?

10.   What development and changes would you like to see in the roles and role relationship you have described above?

C.   MANPOWER DEVELOPMENT

In this section the Committee would like to have your views on how those who work with the mentally handicapped are trained. It is interested in your assessment of the aims and objectives of training courses, their form, including sequence, their content and duration and asks you to refer to the following:

(a)   the initial training of new staff

(b)   the re-training of existing staff

(c)   the continuing professional training of staff *at all levels*

(d)   training opportunities offered to parents and families.

11.   (a)   How appropriate and adequate is the *present* training for the tasks and roles described above of

(i)   Nurses for the mentally handicapped?

(ii)   Residential care staff within local authorities and hospital services?

(iii)   Staff of voluntary agencies?

(iv)   Other staff in regular contact with mentally handicapped people?

(b)   What in your view should be the *future* training, preparation and experience of those responsible for the academic and practical training of staff?

(c)   How appropriate and adequate are the mainstream Brigg's proposals* for the training of nurses who will care for the mentally handicapped and the CCETSW proposals† for the training of residential care staff?

(d)   What changes would *you* propose in both academic and practical training?

(e)   How much training could be "common core" between other health, social services and education staff?

(f)   Where should training courses be based and how should they be organised?

(g)   Can you identify training resources in society which are not being used and could be used?

12.   What are the implications of your proposals in all the preceding sections for career structures and movement?

13.   What are the implications of your proposals for

(a)   the retention of staff?

(b)   for the recruitment of staff;

---

*"Report of the Committee on Nursing" Cmnd 5115 published by HMSO.

†"Residential work is part of social work" CCETSW Paper 3 published by Central Council for Education and Training in Social Work.

D. ORGANISATION OF SERVICES

14. In the light of your evidence, what kind of changes in the *overall* organisation of services, if any, is required

(a) In the short term?

(b) In the long term?

E. ADDITIONAL COMMENTS

15. Are there any additional comments you wish to make?

The main principles on which current thinking about mental handicap at the time of the White Paper was based can be summarised as follows:

(i) A family with a handicapped member has the same needs for general social services as all other families. The family and the handicapped child or adult also need special additional help, which varies according to the severity of the handicap, whether there are associated physical handicaps or behaviour problems, the age of the handicapped person and his family situation.

(ii) Mentally handicapped children and adults should not be segregated unnecessarily from other people of similar age, nor from the general life of the local community.

(iii) Full use should be made of available knowledge which can help to prevent mental handicap or to reduce the severity of its effects.

(iv) There should be a comprehensive initial assessment and periodic reassessment of the needs of each handicapped person and his family.

(v) Each handicapped person needs stimulation, social training and education and purposeful occupation or employment in order to develop to his maximum capacity and to exercise all the skills he acquires, however limited they may be.

(vi) Each handicapped person should live with his own family as long as this does not impose an undue burden on them or him, and he and his family should receive full advice and support. If he has to leave home for a foster home, residential home or hospital, temporarily or permanently, links with his own family should normally be maintained.

(vii) The range of services in every area should be such that the family can be sure that their handicapped member will be properly cared for when it becomes necessary for him to leave the family home.

(viii) When a handicapped person has to leave his family home, temporarily or permanently, the substitute home should be as homelike as possible, even if it is also a hospital. It should provide sympathetic and constant human relationships.

(ix) There should be proper co-ordination in the application of relevant professional skills for the benefit of individual handicapped people and their families, and in the planning and administration of relevant services, whether or not these cross administrative frontiers.

(x) Local authority personal social services for the mentally handicapped should develop as an integral part of the services recently brought together under the Local Authority Social Services Act, 1970.

(xi) There should be close collaboration between these services and those provided by other local authority departments (eg child health services and education), and with general practitioners, hospitals and other services for the disabled.

164

(xii)   Hospital services for the mentally handicapped should be easily accessible to the population they serve. They should be associated with other hospital services, so that a full range of specialist skills is easily available when needed for assessment or treatment.

(xiii)   Hospital and local authority services should be planned and operated in partnership; the Government's proposals for the reorganisation of the National Health Service will encourage the closest co-operation.

(xiv)   Voluntary service can make a contribution to the welfare of mentally handicapped people and their families at all stages of their lives and wherever they are living.

(xv)   Understanding and help from friends and neighbours and from the community at large are needed to help the family to maintain a normal social life and to give the handicapped member as nearly normal a life as his handicap or handicaps permit.

LIST OF INDIVIDUALS AND BODIES WHO SUBMITTED EVIDENCE

*Denotes individuals or bodies submitting oral as well as written evidence
†Denotes individuals or bodies submitting oral evidence only

Miss J Abel
Miss J M Adams
Mrs G Adamson
Mr C Adcroft
Airedale Health District – Senior Nursing Staff
Mr A M Alaszewski
Mr J E Allen
Mr P Allen
Mr C Andrew
Mr J M Andrews
Mr R Antras
Argyll and Clyde Health Board
Mr C and Mrs S A Armitage
Mrs J Armstrong
Miss D Arnold
Assistant Masters Association
Association of Assistant Mistresses – Members
†Association of British Paediatric Nurses
*Association of County Councils
Association of Directors of Social Services
†Association of District Councils
Association of Hospital and Residential Care Officers
†Association of Metropolitan Authorities
*Association of Nurse Administrators
†Association of Nurse Administrators (Wales)
*Association of Professions for the Mentally Handicapped
Association of Psychiatric Nurse Tutors (Scotland)
Associations of Head Mistresses and Nurse Administrators (Joint Committee)
Avon Area Health Authority – Senior Nursing Staff
Avon County Council– Social Services Department
Aycliffe Hospital – Nursing Staff

Mr K Baker
†Dr Barnardo's Homes
Mrs P Barnsley
Mr D F Barton
Bedfordshire Area Health Authority
Berkshire Area Health Authority
Berkshire County Council (Social Services Department) – Senior Mental Handicap
   Hostel Staff
Birmingham Metropolitan District Council and Area Health Authority – Joint Con-
   sultative Committee
Mr E J Botley
Botleys Park Hospital – Nursing Staff
Mr A C Bowden and Mr D O Mole
Mr J Bradbury and Mr K W Cokayne
Mr C Branchflower
Brentry Hospital – Occupational Therapy Department
Brighton Health District – Nursing Staff

British Association for Behavioural Psychotherapy
British Association of the Hard of Hearing—Social Services Committee
*British Association of Occupational Therapists
British Association of Occupational Therapists (Scottish Committee)
British Association of Psychotherapists
*British Association of Social Workers
*British Medical Association
British Medical Association (Scottish Office) – Scottish Joint Consultants Committee
*British Paediatric Association
British Paedodontic Society
*British Psychological Society
British Psychological Society (Clinical Division) – North East Midlands Branch
Brockhall Hospital – Nursing Staff
Bromham Hospital – Nursing Staff
Bromham Hospital – Senior Nursing Staff
Bromley Community Health Council
Broughton Hospital – Multi-disciplinary Staff
Bryn-y-Neuadd Hospital – Nursing Staff
Bryn-y-Neuadd Hospital – Parent/Relative Staff Association
Bryn-y-Neuadd Hospital – Student and Pupil Nurses
Mrs W A Burley
Mrs M Burns
Bury Area Health Authority – Multi-disciplinary Working Group
Bury St Edmunds Health District – Mental Handicap Nursing Liaison Group
Cambridgeshire Area Health Authority
Camden and Islington Area Health Authority and London Boroughs of Camden and
    Islington – Joint Consultative Committee
*Campaign for the Mentally Handicapped
Camphill-Rudolf Steiner-Schools
Canterbury and Thanet Health District – Mental Handicap Nursing Staff
Cardiff and Vale of Glamorgan Community Health Councils
'Cardiff Universities Social Services
Mr C Caudle
The Hon Mrs Cawley
Cell Barnes Hospital – Nursing Staff
Cell Barnes Hospital – Student and Pupil Nurses
'Central Council for Education and Training in Social work
Central Health District (Manchester) – Health Visitors
Central Nottinghamshire Health District
Mrs E Chadwick
Miss J Chapman
Charles Frears School of Nursing – Psychiatric Department
Mr C P Charlesworth
*Chartered Society Of Physiotherapy
Chelmsley Hospital – Nursing Staff
Cheshire Area Health Authority
Cheshire Area Health Authority – Area Nurses and Midwives Advisory Committee
Cheshire Area Health Authority – Area Team of Officers
Mrs S Chilton
Mr D Clark
Mr R Clarke
Mr T Clay
Mrs J Clemente
Cleveland County Council – Social Services Department
Coed-Du Hospital – Nursing Staff
Coldeast Hospital – Group of Nursing Staff

Coldharbour Hospital – Report of Multi-disciplinary Symposium
Coleshill Hall Hospital – Nursing Staff
Committee for Clinical Nursing Studies
Committee of Parents Against Substandard Subnormality Institutions or Nursing (COMPASSION)
*Confederation of Health Service Employees
Confederation of Health Service Employees (Forest Hospital Branch)
Mr E B Connors
Convention of Scottish Local Authorities
Mr D T H Cook
Mr P Corbett
Miss J N Corley
*Cornwall and Isles of Scilly Area Health Authority – Multi-disciplinary Working Party
Dr D Cortazzi
Cottage and Rural Enterprises Ltd (CARE)
Mr N Coulson
Council for the Education and Training of Health Visitors
Coventry Metropolitan District – Social Services Department
Mr R Cowan
Dr M J Craft
Dr R D G Creery
Mr P Creighton
Crewe Health District – Psychiatric Division
Mr W Crosbie

Dale Centre, Lanark – Staff
Darenth Park Hospital – Activities Team
Darenth Park Hospital – Staff Working Party
Darlington Community Health Council
Dartford and Gravesham Community Health Council – Mental Handicap Working Party
Mr R E Davis
Dean Hill Hospital – Nursing Staff
Miss A Denholm
Derbyshire Area Health Authority – Area Nursing and Midwifery Committee
Derbyshire County Council (Social Services Department) – Senior Management Team Group
Miss P N Devine
Devon County Council – Social Services and Education Departments
Ms H I S Dewar
Dingleton Hospital – Multi-disciplinary Group of Staff
Doncaster Area Health Authority – Mental Handicap Nursing Staff
Doncaster Metropolitan Borough – Social Services Department
Mr T A Donnelly
Mrs C J Dorrington
Dovenby Hall Hospital – Working Party
Dudley Metropolitan Borough – Social Services Department
Dundee Health District (Psychiatric Services) – Division of Psychiatry
Durham Area Health Authority – Area Nursing and Midwifery Committee
Durham County Council – Social Services Department
Mr and Mrs R A Dyson

Earls House Hospital – Nursing Staff
East Anglian Regional Health Authority – Regional Nurse Training Committee
East Cumbria Health District – Health Visitors
East Hertfordshire Community Health Council

East Sussex Area Health Authority
East Sussex County Council (Social Services Department) – Hove Division Working Party
Eastbourne Community Health Council
Eastbourne Health District – Multi-disciplinary Staff
Mr C J Eastwood
Educational Institute of Scotland
Edward Lawson Adult Training Centre, Wishaw – Staff
Mr D Ellis
Essex County Council – Social Services Department

Dr A C Fairburn
Family Planning Association – Education Unit
Mr P J Farrell and Mr H S K Lee
Mr M F Fenn
Fieldhead Hospital – Nursing Staff
Fife Health Board – Area Nursing and Midwifery Consultative Committee
Fife Regional Council – Social Work Committee
Mr H Firth
Mr J B and Mrs P A Fitton
Mr W P Fitzgerald
Mr G Folland
Mr G K Forbes
Dr J A S Forman
Dr I A Fraser
Miss M Fraser Gamble
Mr B Freeman
Frenchay Health District – Mental Handicap Sector Management Team
*Friends of South Ockendon Hospital Association

Ellen Gallagher
Mrs S H Gardner
Mr G D Garioch
Mr K Garnett
Mr C E Gathercole
Mr M Gee
*General Nursing Council for England and Wales
*General Nursing Council for Scotland
Mr R H Genge
Mrs J Gessler
Mr M S Gibberd
Dr J Gibson
Mr M J Gifford
Gloucestershire Area Health Authority
Gloucestershire Area Health Authority – Area Nursing and Midwifery Committee
Gloucestershire Area Health Authority – Health Care Planning Team for Mental Handicap
Gloucestershire County Council – Social Services Department
Gogarburn Hospital – Multi-disciplinary Staff Groups
Gogarburn Hospital – Physiotherapy Department
Gogarburn Hospital – Psychology Department
Gogarburn Hospital (Children's Unit) – Nursing and Psychology Staff

169

Mr P Goodchild
Mr F Goodwin
*Mr V Gorman
Mr G W B Grant
Greater Glasgow Health Board – Mental Health Programme Planning Committee
    Sub-group
Greaves Hall Hospital – Nursing Staff
Miss V M Greenham
Mr R Grier
Group of Social Workers, S.E. London and Kent
Group of Social Workers (Employment), Bristol
Mrs E A Gutteridge
Guy's Community Health Council
Gwent Area Health Authority – Area Nursing and Midwifery Advisory Committee

Mr J V Hackett
Dr S S Hadi
Hamilton/East Kilbride Health District – District Executive Group
Mr J Hammett
Hampshire County Council – Social Services Department
Hanham Hall Hospital – Nursing Staff
Mr S Hardy
Harmston Hall and Caistor Hospitals – Nursing Staff and Caistor Parents Association
Dr G F Harris
Mr R Harrison-Boyle
Hastings Community Health Council
Hastings Health District – Nursing Staff
Mr D N Hay
Health Visitors' Association
Dr J R Hegarty
Henchard House, Dorchester – Staff
Hensol Hospital – Nursing Staff
Hereford and Worcester County Council – Social Services Department
Hertfordshire Area Health Authority (Dacorum Division) – Health Visiting and
    District Nursing Staff
Hertfordshire Area Health Authority (St Albans Division) – Community Health
    Services
Hertfordshire County Council – Social Services Department
Mr J G Hindle
Mr B E Hodges
Mr D Hodgson
Dr J Hogg
Mr J Hook
Hortham Hospital (Nurse Training School) – Teaching Staff
Mr D L Hughes
Mr J Hughes
Mr S G Hughes
Hull Health District (Division of Mental Handicap) – Nursing Staff
Mr G and Mr J Hulme
Elizabeth Hunter
Margaret Hutchinson

Ida Darwin Hospital – Clinical Services Advisory Committee
Ida Darwin Hospital – Nursing Staff
Mr T Ingham

Inner London Education Authority
Institute of Health Service Administrators
Institute of Home Help Organisers

Jane Walker Hospital – Nursing Staff
Mrs C Jones
Mr E J Jones
†Professor K Jones and Mr J Brown
Miss M B Jones

Mr S G Kelly
Kensington and Chelsea and Westminster Area Health Authority – Area Nursing and
    Midwifery Advisory Committee
Kent Area Health Authority – Area Nursing and Midwifery Committee
Mrs Kerr
Kidderminster Community Health Council – Mental Subnormality Working Party
Mrs U Kiernan
Mr J A E Kiley
King's Community Health Council – Executive Committee
King's Health District – Mental Handicap Working Party
Mr H W Knight

Mr B M Lambert
Lanarkshire Health Board – Auxiliary Association
Lanarkshire Health Board – Area Nursing and Midwifery Advisory Committee Sub-
    committee
L'Arche Ltd
Lea Castle Hospital – Nursing Staff
Lea Hospital – Nursing Staff
League of Friends of Prudhoe Hospital
*Leavesden Group of Senior Nursing Managers
Mrs M Lee
Mr S A Lee
Leeds Metropolitan District – Department of Education
Leeds Metropolitan District – Social Services Department
Leeds Community Health Councils
Leicestershire Area Health Authority – Group of Psychologists
*Leicestershire Area Health Authority – Senior Nurse Managers and Ward Staff
Mrs C Leith
Lenham Hospital – Nursing Staff
Lennox Castle Hospital – Nursing Staff
Mr J Lewis
Lewisham Health District – Community Nursing Staff
Lewisham Health District – Nursing Staff
Lewisham Community Health Council
Leybourne Grange Hospital – Medical Committee
Miss M Ling
Mrs M Littlewood
Liverpool Area Health Authority – Multi-disciplinary Ad Hoc Working Party
Liverpool Catholic Children's and Social Services
Llanfrechfa Grange Hospital – Multi-disciplinary Working Party
London Borough of Brent – Social Services Department
London Borough of Bromley
London Borough of Camden

171

London Borough of Enfield (Social Services Department) – Working Party of Officers
London Borough of Greenwich
London Borough of Hammersmith – Social Services Department
London Borough of Hillingdon – Education and Social Services Committees
London Borough of Lewisham (Social Services Department) – Social Services Staff
London Borough of Newham (Social Services Department) – Working Party
London Borough of Tower Hamlets – Social Services Committee
London Borough of Waltham Forest – Education and Social Services Departments
London Borough of Wandsworth (Social Services Department) – Care Services Division
Mr E C Long
Lothian Health Board
Lothian Health Board – Area Dental Committee
Lothian Health Board – Area Nursing and Midwifery Committee
Lothian Health Board – Occupational, Speech and Physiotherapy Staff
Mr T S Lyne

Mrs A L McCallum
Mr S McCamley
Mr J S MacCarthy
Mr C R McDade
Mrs J McDonald
Mr J McFadden
Mrs M A McKeane
Dr W McKee
Mr F McKendry
Dr T F MacKintosh
Mr B H McLaren
Mr E J McMahon and Mr A Pugh
Maidstone Community Health Council
Mr C Manby
Manchester Metropolitan District (Social Services Department) – Working Group of Staff
Mr E Marchant
Mr G Marsden
Mrs J Marshall
Dr R H Martin
Mr D R Matthews
Mr A E May
Meanwood Park Hospital – Nursing Staff
Dr M R Mellor
Mentally Handicapped Children's Aid Society (Ashton-under-Lyne and District)
Merton, Sutton and Wandsworth Area Health Authority (Area Nursing and Midwifery Committee) – Nursing Working Party
Mid-Glamorgan County Council
Mr T Miller
Miss K Mogford
Monyhull Hospital – Social Work Staff
Monyhull Hospital – Working Party
Pauline Morgan
Motherwell/Lanark Health District – Consultant Psychiatrist (Child Psychiatry)
Motherwell/Lanark Health District – Consultant Psychiatrist (Mental Deficiency)
Mrs S M Moulton
Mrs E F Muir
Mrs J Murray

172

Mr H K Naghen
National and Local Government Officers Association
*National Association for Mental Health (MIND)
†National Association for Mental Health (MIND, Wales)
*National Association for the Welfare of Children in Hospital
National Association for the Welfare of Children in Hospital (York Branch)
*National Association of Teachers of the Mentally Handicapped
National Children's Home
National Council of Social Service – National Organisations Division
*National Nursery Examination Board
National Society for Autistic Children
*National Society For Mentally Handicapped Children
†National Union of Public Employees
National Union of Teachers
Mr P E Nesbitt
Newcastle Area Health Authority – Division of Psychiatry
Mrs K Newman
Norah Fry Hospital – Nursing Staff
Norfolk Area Health Authority – Area Nursing and Midwifery Committee
Norfolk County Council – Social Services Department
North Derbyshire Community Health Council
North Derbyshire Health District – Multi-disciplinary Team
North East Thames Regional Health Authority – Working Party of Nurses
North Eastern Area Nurse Training Committee, Scotland
North Lothian Health District – Nursing Staff
North West Thames Regional Health Authority
North Western Regional Health Authority
Northamptonshire County Council (Social Services Department) – Residential Care
    Staff
Northern Health District (Sheffield) – Multi-disciplinary Team for the Mentally
    Handicapped
Northern Ireland Council for Nurses and Midwives
Northern Regional Health Authority – Consultant Psychiatrists in Mental Handicap
Northgate Hospital – Local Management Team
Northumberland and North Tyneside Area Health Authorities – Multi-disciplinary
    Group
Norwich Community Health Council – Mental Health Committee
*Norwich Health District (Mental Handicap Division) – Working Party
Nottinghamshire Area Health Authority – Area Nursing and Midwifery Advisory
    Committee
Nottinghamshire County Council

Offerton House Hospital – Nursing Staff
Josephine Orchard
Mr M O'Reilly

Dr D N Parfitt
Mrs M Parrick and Mr P Dugdale
Mr D W Penfold
Dr D J Pereira Gray
Miss E Phillips
Mair Pierce
Dr T L Pilkington
Pollockshields, Killearn St, South Portland St and Whiteinch Adult Training Centres
    and Work Centre – Staff

Powys Health Authority
Pre-school Play Groups Association (Special Needs Committee) – Sub-committee on Handicap
Mr W K Prestwich
Princess Marina Hospital – Staff Working Group
Priorsdale Hostel, Jesmond – Staff
Prison Officers Association
Prudhoe Hospital – Nursing Staff

*Mr C J P Quigley
Dr M Quinn

Elizabeth A Reed
Dr T W Rees
*Residential Care Association – National Standing Committees for Mental Handicap and Mental Health
Residential Hostel, 223 Old Shoreham Rd, Portslade – Residential Staff
Mrs N Roberts
Rochdale Area Health Authority – Area Nursing and Midwifery Committee
Rochdale Metropolitan Borough – Social Services Department
Mr S Roe
Mr J W M Rookes
Mr P J Rookes
Rotherham Metropolitan Borough – Social Services Department
*Royal College of Nursing of the United Kingdom
Royal College of Nursing of the United Kingdom (Prudhoe Hospital Branch)
Royal College of Nursing of the United Kingdom (Scottish Board)
Royal College of Physicians of Edinburgh
*Royal College of Psychiatrists
Royal College of Psychiatrists (Scottish Division) – Mental Deficiency Section
*Royal College of Psychiatrists (Welsh Division) – Executive Committee and Sub-normality Section
Royal Colleges of Physicians of the United Kingdom – Faculty of Community Medicine
Royal Earlswood Hospital – Nursing Staff
Royal Earlswood Hospital – Technical and Social Training Staff
Royal National Institute for the Deaf
Royal Scottish National Hospital
Royal Scottish National Hospital – Nursing Staff
Royal Western Counties Hospital Group – Nursing Staff
Royal Western Counties Hospital Group – Student Nurses
Mr T Ryan

St Catherine's Hospital – Multi-disciplinary Working Group
St Clement's Hospital – Mental Handicap Nursing Staff
St Joseph's Hospital – Multi-disciplinary Staff
St Lawrence's Hospital – Professional Consultative Committee
St Lawrence's Hospital – Senior Nurses and Head Social Worker
St Peter's Hospital (Crossman Unit) – Nursing Staff
St Thomas' Health District – Mental Handicap Health Care Planning Team
Salford Area Health Authority
Salop County Council – Social Services Department
Muriel J Sanders
Sandwell Metropolitan Borough
Mrs S Sapsed
Mr D T Savage

174

Scottish Association of Nurse Administrators
Scottish District Nursing Association
Scottish Education Department
Scottish Education Department – Social Work Services Group
Scottish Health Service Planning Council – National Nursing and Midwifery
     Consultative Committee
Sefton Metropolitan Borough – Social Services Department
Mr I R Semple
Mr R Semrock
Mr E Shannon
Sheffield Area Health Authority – Nursing Staff
Sheffield Metropolitan District (Social Services Department) – The Special Interest
     Group
Mrs M Shepherd
Mr P Short
Mr A M Smith
Mr J P Smith
Society of Chiropodists
South Birmingham Health District – Health Care Planning Team for Mental Handicap
South Derbyshire Community Health Council
South Gwent Community Health Council
South Nottingham Health District – Community Nursing Staff
South Ockendon Hospital – Medical Committee
South Ockendon Hospital – Nursing Staff
South West Thames Regional Health Authority (Medical and Nursing and Midwifery
     Committees) – Joint Working Party
Southmead Community Health Council
Southmead Health District – Mental Handicap Staff
*Spastics Society
Dr D A Spencer
Mrs J M Stanger
Mr K Stanley
Mrs G M Stephens
Dr J B P Stephenson
Stoke Park Group of Hospitals – Nursing Staff
Stoke Park Group of Hospitals – Occupational Therapy Staff
Stoke Park Group of Hospitals – Physiotherapy Staff
Stoke Park Group of Hospitals – Speech Therapy Staff
Ruth M Stone
Mrs J C Stormonth Darling
Strathclyde Regional Council (Department of Social Work) – Social Work Staff
Dr M K Strelling
Mr W Stuttard
Surrey Area Health Authority (Area Medical Committee) – Consultants in Mental
     Handicap Sub-group
Mr A H Sutherland
Professor J N Swallow
Swindon Health District – Nursing Staff

Tameside Metropolitan Borough – Social Services Department
Mr J Taylor
Mr J H Taylor
Mrs J M Taylor
Tayside Health Board – Area Nursing and Midwifery Committee
Tayside Health Board – Senior Nursing Staff
The Cheshire Home for Mentally Handicapped Children – Management Committee

The Close Hostel, Sunderland – Staff
The Forest Hospital – Nursing Staff
The Hospital for Sick Children – Board of Governors
*The Manor Hospital – Nursing Staff
The Manor Hospital – Project by Student Nurses
W/S Thomas
Dr I G Thomson
Thornton Lodge Hospital – Nursing and Professional Staff
Dr J G Thorpe
Mrs A J Tierney
Mrs J Titley
Todmorden Hospitals – Nursing Staff
Mr D M Torpy
Tower Hamlets Health District
Mr J N Towler
Trafford Borough Council – Social Services Department
Trent Regional Health Authority
Trent Regional Health Authority Conference Centre – Group of Nurses on Study
    Course
Mr F and Mrs G Trevers
Miss M A Twohig

Mr E T Udall
United Kingdom Council for Overseas Student Affairs
University of London (Institute of Child Health) – Wolfson Centre Staff

Mr J Varley

Walsall Nursing Advisory Committee
Miss B Walsh
Dr R M Walters
Frances M Warner
Warwickshire Area Health Authority
Warwickshire Area Health Authority – Area Nurses and Midwives Professional
    Advisory Committee
Warwickshire County Council – Social Services Committee
Mr D A and Mrs S A Waskett
Dr M E Watkins
Dr M Way
Mrs P Webb
Mr C Webster
*Wessex Health Care Evaluation Research Team
Wessex Regional Health Authority – District Nursing Officer
West Berkshire Health District (Mental Handicap Division) – Nursing Staff
West Central Area Nurse Training Committee, Scotland
West Glamorgan Area Health Authority
West Lothian Health District – Community Nursing Staff
West Midlands Regional Health Authority – Senior Nursing Staff
West Somerset Health District (District Management Team) – Multi-disciplinary
    Working Party
Dr B P Westworth
Mr N J Whaley
Whittington Hall Hospital – Nursing Staff
Dr C E Williams

176

Mr J C Williams
Mr P Williams
*Dr B Winokur
Wirral Area Health Authority
Mr J B Wood
Dr G E Woods
Mr G Worrall

Mr F Yates
Mr C Young

LIST OF PLACES VISITED BY MEMBERS OF THE COMMITTEE

Astbury House Hostel, Birmingham

Balderton Hospital, Newark
Beachcroft Unit, Oakwood Hall Hospital, Rotherham
Borocourt Hospital, Reading
Broad Oaks Home, Nottingham
Brockhall Hospital, Blackburn
Brothers of Charity Residential and Day Centre, St Aidan's, Melrose
Broughton Hospital, Chester

Calderhouse House Hostel, Padiham
Calderstones Hospital, Nr Blackburn
Camphill Village Trust, Aberdeen
Castle Priory College, Wallingford
Causeway Green Adult Training Centre, Warley
Cavendish House Hostel, Workington
Cefndy Hostel, Rhyl
Churchill House Hospital, Bracknell

Delph Manor Hostel, Leeds
Dilkes Wood Adult Training Centre, South Ockendon
Distington Adult Training Centre, Workington
Dovenby Hall Hospital, Cockermouth

Elmtree Road Group Home, Maltby

Fairmile House, Christchurch
Family Group Home, Tapley Avenue, Wrexham

Gogarburn Hospital, Edinburgh
Greenacres Hostel, Sheffield

Havering Technical College
Henchard House, Dorchester
Henley Hostel, Kettering
Henllan Adult Training Centre, Nr Denbigh
Henllan Hostel, Nr Denbigh

Kettering Industrial Unit

Leighton View, Sheffield
Leybourne Grange Hospital, West Malling
Lightwood House, Sheffield

Maltby Adult Training Centre
Meanwood Park Hospital, Leeds

Nichols Centre Adult Training Centre, Exeter
Nichols Centre Residential Care Unit, Exeter
Northcroft Hostel, Bracknell

Parkhill Lodge Hostel, Maltby
Princess Marina Hospital, Northampton

Queen Mary's Hospital for Children, Carshalton

Raeden Assessment Centre, Aberdeen
Rampton Special Hospital, Retford
Rosehill Adult Training Centre, Aberdeen
Rothwell Adult Training Centre, Leeds
Royal Western Counties Hospitals, Starcross
Rusthall Elms Adult Training Centre, Tunbridge Wells
Rusthall Elms Hostel – Tunbridge Wells
Ryegate Day Care Centre, Sheffield

St Margaret's Hospital, Birmingham
South Ockendon Hospital, Essex
Springbank Adult Training Centre, Padiham
Springwood Adult Training Centre, Nottingham
Stockport College of Technology
Strafford House, Sheffield

The Cherries Group Home, Slough
Tree Tops Special Care Unit, Exeter

Westwood House, Southampton
Whiteacre Hostel, Thurrock
Winchester House Hostel, Elgin
Windlesford Green Hostel, Leeds
Woodlands Hospital, Aberdeen
Woodside Lane Assessment Centre, Sheffield

GLOSSARY OF TERMS USED IN THE REPORT

ATC — Adult Training Centre, providing social and work training, and further education for mentally handicapped adults.

Briggs Report — The Report of the Committee on Nursing chaired by Professor Asa Briggs.

Care Assistant — A qualified or (more usually) unqualified worker in a local authority residential home.

Care Worker — Our proposed new worker providing residential care to mentally handicapped people living in mental handicap homes and hospitals.

CCETSW — The Central Council for Education and Training in Social Work.

CQSW — The Certificate of Qualification in Social Work; the qualifying training for social workers.

CRSW — The Certificate in Residential Social Work; a training course for residential social workers, now being replaced by the CQSW and the CSS.

CRCCYP/SCRCCYP — The Certificate (or Senior Certificate) in the Residential Care of Children and Young People; a training course for residential social workers working with children and young people, now being replaced by the CQSW and the CSS.

CSS — The Certificate in Social Service; a new form of training for a range of staff groups in the personal social services.

Dip TMHA — The Diploma in the Training and Further Education of Mentally Handicapped Adults; the training course for ATC Instructors and Managers, now being replaced by the CSS.

Group Home — Unstaffed residential accommodation, with or without support services, for a small group of mentally handicapped adults.

GNC — General Nursing Council; there are two Councils, one for England and Wales and one for Scotland.

Nursing Assistant — An unqualified worker assisting the nurses in a mental handicap hospital.

OPCS — Office of Population Censuses and Surveys.

Pupil — A learner undergoing training for the Roll of Nurses.

Register — The Register of Nurses kept by the General Nursing Councils.

Registered nurses:

SRN — State Registered Nurse (RGN – Registered General Nurse in Scotland);

RMN — Registered Mental Nurse;

RNMS — Registered Nurse for the Mentally Subnormal (RMND – Registered Nurse for Mental Defectives in Scotland);

180

RSCN	— Registered Sick Children's Nurse;
Roll	— The Roll of Nurses kept by the General Nursing Councils.
Enrolled nurses:	
SEN	— State Enrolled Nurse (Enrolled Nurse in Scotland);
	— Senior Enrolled Nurse;
SEN(M)	— State Enrolled Mental Nurse;
SEN(MS)	— State Enrolled Nurse for the Mentally Subnormal. (The Roll in Scotland is not divided.)
Sheffield Method	— Method of calculating staff/resident ratios used in the DHSS Sheffield Development Project.
Structure:	— Our proposed new staffing structure for care workers in the NHS and local authorities.
Basic Care Worker	— A first level in-service trained care worker;
Trainee	— A learner taking the qualifying training;
Qualified Care Worker	— A worker on the first qualified level who has taken the qualifying training;
Advanced (Unit) Care Worker	— A qualified and experienced worker based in a living Unit;
Unit Head	— A qualified care worker in charge of a living Unit;
Advanced (Management) Care Worker	— A qualified and experienced worker not based in a living Unit, with advisory and management responsibilities;
Senior Manager	— A qualified and experienced care worker responsible for policy planning across a range of client groups or services.
Student	— A learner undergoing training for the Register of Nurses.
Unit	— A Unit of staffed residential accommodation for mentally handicapped people; a living Unit may be a self-contained home, a ward in a hospital, or a sub-group of people living in a ward or home.
Ward	— A Unit of residential accommodation for mentally handicapped people within a hospital comprising sleeping and day space.
White Paper	— The 1971 White Paper "Better Services for the Mentally Handicapped".

181

LIST OF REFERENCES IN THE REPORT

(Paragraph numbers at the end of each reference refer to this Report.)

1. DEPARTMENT OF HEALTH AND SOCIAL SECURITY, SCOTTISH HOME AND HEALTH DEPARTMENT AND WELSH OFFICE. *Report of the Committee on Nursing.* Chairman: Professor Asa Briggs. Cmnd 5115. HMSO. London. 1972. (Paragraph 1.)

2. DEPARTMENT OF HEALTH AND SOCIAL SECURITY AND WELSH OFFICE. *Better Services for the Mentally Handicapped.* Cmnd 4683. HMSO. London. 1971. (Paragraphs 3, 88.)

3. KUSHLICK, A. The Prevalence of Recognised Mental Subnormality. *Copenhagen Conference Strides in Mental Retardation.* 12:550–556. 1964. (Paragraph 11.)

4. WING, J K and FRYERS, T. *Psychiatric Services in Camberwell and Salford, Statistics from the Camberwell and Salford Registers 1964–1974.* 1975. (Paragraph 11.)

5. MARTINDALE, A. *Sheffield Case Register Report No. 1.* 1975. (Paragraph 11.)

6. DEPARTMENT OF HEALTH AND SOCIAL SECURITY AND WELSH OFFICE. *Census of Mentally Handicapped Patients in Hospital in England and Wales at the end of 1970.* HMSO. London. 1972. (Paragraph 12.)

7. DEPARTMENT OF HEALTH AND SOCIAL SECURITY AND WELSH OFFICE. *The Census of Residential Accommodation: 1970.* HMSO. London. 1972. (Paragraph 12.)

8. JONES, K. *A History of the Mental Health Services.* Routledge and Kegan Paul. London. 1972. (Paragraph 21.)

9. TODD, F J. *Social Work with the Mentally Subnormal.* Routledge and Kegan Paul. London. 1967. (Paragraph 24.)

10. ROYAL COMMISSION ON THE LAW RELATING TO MENTAL ILLNESS AND MENTAL DEFICIENCY, 1954–1957. *Report.* Cmnd 169. HMSO. London 1957. (Paragraph 25.)

11. MINISTRY OF HEALTH. *A National Health Service.* Cmnd 6502. HMSO. London. 1944. (Paragraph 25.)

12. GRIFFITHS, O. *A Report on Mental and Mental Deficiency Hospitals 1949.* General Nursing Council for England and Wales. (Unpublished.) (Paragraph 28.)

13. SCOTTISH HOME AND HEALTH DEPARTMENT. *The Health Service in Scotland: The Way Ahead.* HMSO. Edinburgh. 1976. (Paragraph 31.)

14. MINISTRY OF HEALTH. *Report of the Working Party on Social Workers in the Local Authority Health and Welfare Services.* Chairman: Miss Eileen L Younghusband, CBE, LLD, JP. HMSO. London. 1959. (Paragraph 32.)

15. HOME OFFICE, DEPARTMENT OF EDUCATION AND SCIENCE, MINISTRY OF HOUSING AND LOCAL GOVERNMENT AND MINISTRY OF HEALTH. *Report of the Committee on Local Authority and Allied Personal Social Services.* Chairman: Frederic Seebohm Esq. Cmnd 3703. HMSO. London. 1968. (Paragraph 32.)

16. MINISTRY OF HEALTH. *A Hospital Plan for England and Wales.* Cmnd 1604. HMSO. London. 1962. (Paragraph 35.)

17. MINISTRY OF HEALTH. *The Development of Community Care.* Cmnd 1973. HMSO. London. 1964. (Paragraph 35.)

18. MINISTRY OF HEALTH. *National Health Service. Improving the Effectiveness of the Hospital Service for the Mentally Subnormal.* HM(65)104. Ministry of Health. London. 1965. (Paragraph 35.)

19. DEPARTMENT OF HEALTH AND SOCIAL SECURITY. *Report of the Committee of Inquiry into Allegations of Ill-Treatment of Patients and Other Irregularities at the Ely Hospital, Cardiff.* Chairman: Mr Geoffrey Howe, QC. Cmnd 3975. HMSO. London. 1969. (Paragraph 36.)

20. MINISTRY OF HEALTH. *Interim Measures to Improve Hospital Services for the Mentally Handicapped.* Paper for Regional Hospital Board Chairmen 10/69. Ministry of Health. London. 1969. (Paragraph 36.)

21. NATIONAL DEVELOPMENT GROUP FOR THE MENTALLY HANDICAPPED. *Helping Mentally Handicapped People in Hospital.* HMSO. London. 1978. (Paragraphs 38, 334.)

22. DEPARTMENT OF HEALTH AND SOCIAL SECURITY, HOME OFFICE, WELSH OFFICE AND LORD CHANCELLOR'S DEPARTMENT. *Review of the Mental Health Act, 1959.* Cmnd 7320. HMSO. London. 1958. (Paragraph 38.)

23. UNITED NATIONS GENERAL ASSEMBLY. *Declaration on the Rights of Mentally Retarded Persons.* Resolution 2856, 26th Session, 1972. (Paragraph 88.)

24. LONDON BOROUGH OF WANDSWORTH. *Project 74: A Research Study in which Mentally Handicapped People Speak for Themselves.* Social Services Department, Research and Planning Section. 1976. (Paragraph 130.)

25. BAYLEY, M. *Mental Handicap and Community Care.* Routledge and Kegan Paul. London. 1973. (Paragraph 131.)

26. NATIONAL DEVELOPMENT GROUP FOR THE MENTALLY HANDICAPPED. *Day Services for Mentally Handicapped Adults.* Pamphlet No. 5. HMSO. London. 1977. (Paragraph 132.)

27. KING, R D, RAYNES, N V and TIZARD, J. *Patterns of Residential Care.* Routledge and Kegan Paul. London. 1971. (Paragraphs 138, 151.)

28. KUSHLICK, A, FELCE, D, PALMER, J and SMITH, J. *Evidence to the Committee of Inquiry into Mental Handicap Nursing and Care from the Health Care Evaluation Research Team, Winchester.* HCERT. Winchester. 1976. (Paragraph 150.)

29. OSWIN, M. *Children Living in Long-Stay Hospitals.* Spastics International Medical Publication. London. 1978. (Paragraphs 152, 185, 334, 377.)

30. JONES, K. *Opening the Door.* Routledge and Kegan Paul. London. 1975. (Paragraphs 152, 375.)

31. DEPARTMENT OF HEALTH AND SOCIAL SECURITY. *Fit for the Future: The Report of the Committee on Child Health Services.* (Chairman: Emeritus Professor S D M Court, CBE, MD, FRCP, FCST.) Cmnd 6684. HMSO. London. 1976. (Paragraphs 159, 311.)

32. GUARDIAN. *Article in The Guardian newspaper.* London. 7 September 1978. (Paragraph 162.)

33. SOCIAL SERVICES LIAISON GROUP. *Residential Care: Staffing and Training.* Report of a Working Party, Chairman: Mr James B Chaplin, CBE. 1978. (Paragraph 169.)

34. RESIDENTIAL CARE ASSOCIATION. *Residential Task in Child Care.* Report of a Study Group Meeting at Castle Priory College. 1972. (Paragraph 169.)

35. DEPARTMENT OF HEALTH AND SOCIAL SECURITY. *Sheffield Development Project Feasibility Study.* Department of Health and Social Security. 1971. (Paragraphs 170, 182.)

36. OFFICE OF POPULATION CENSUSES AND SURVEYS. *Population Projections 1975–2015.* Series PP2, No. 7. HMSO. London. 1977. (Paragraph 203.)

37. DEPARTMENT OF EMPLOYMENT. *Employment Gazette.* Vol. 86, No. 4. HMSO. London. 1978. (Paragraph 203.)

38. DEPARTMENT OF HEALTH AND SOCIAL SECURITY. *Manpower and Training for the Social Services.* Report of a Working Party. Chairman: Mr Robin A Birch. HMSO. London. 1976. (Paragraphs 229, 255, 358.)

39. CENTRAL COUNCIL FOR EDUCATION AND TRAINING IN SOCIAL WORK. *A New Form of Training – The Certificate in Social Service.* Paper 9:1. CCETSW. London. 1975. (Paragraph 231.)

40. CENTRAL COUNCIL FOR EDUCATION AND TRAINING IN SOCIAL WORK. *The Certificate in Social Service – A Guide to Planning.* Paper 9:2. CCETSW. London. 1976. (Paragraphs 243, 250.)

41. CENTRAL COUNCIL FOR EDUCATION AND TRAINING IN SOCIAL WORK. *The Certificate in Social Service – Further Guidance on Planning and Development.* Paper 9:3. CCETSW. London. 1977. (Paragraph 250.)

42. DEPARTMENT OF EDUCATION AND SCIENCE. *The Training of Teachers for Further Education.* Circular 11/77. Department of Education and Science. 1977. (Paragraph 261.)

43. DEPARTMENT OF HEALTH AND SOCIAL SECURITY. *The Role of Psychologists in the Health Services.* Report of the Sub-Committee. (Chairman: Professor W H Trethowan, CBE, FRCP, FRCPsych.) HMSO. London. 1977. (Paragraph 311.)

44. DEPARTMENT OF EDUCATION AND SCIENCE. *Special Educational Needs.* Report of the Committee of Enquiry into the Education of Handicapped Children and Young People. (Chairman: Mrs H M Warnock.) Cmnd 7212. HMSO. London. 1978. (Paragraph 311.)

45. WYNN, M and WYNN, A. *Prevention of Handicap of Perinatal Origin.* Foundation for Education and Research in Childbearing. London. 1976. (Paragraph 342.)

Printed in England for Her Majesty's Stationery Office by Harrison & Sons (London) Ltd.

27544   Dd 294799   K160   2/79